Assembling the Pieces of a Systematic Review

MEDICAL LIBRARY ASSOCIATION BOOKS

The Medical Library Association (MLA) features books that showcase the expertise of health sciences librarians for other librarians and professionals.

MLA Books are excellent resources for librarians in hospitals, medical research practice, and other settings. These volumes will provide health care professionals and patients with accurate information that can improve outcomes and save lives.

Each book in the series has been overseen editorially since conception by the Medical Library Association Books Panel, composed of MLA members with expertise spanning the breadth of health sciences librarianship.

About the Medical Library Association

Founded in 1898, MLA is a 501(c)(3) nonprofit, educational organization of 3,500 individual and institutional members in the health sciences information field that provides lifelong educational opportunities, supports a knowledgebase of health information research, and works with a global network of partners to promote the importance of quality information for improved health to the health care community and the public.

Books in the Series:

The Medical Library Association Guide to Providing Consumer and Patient Health Information edited by Michele Spatz
Health Sciences Librarianship edited by M. Sandra Wood
Curriculum-Based Library Instruction: From Cultivating Faculty Relationships to Assessment edited by Amy Blevins and Megan Inman

Mobile Technologies for Every Library by Ann Whitney Gleason
Marketing for Special and Academic Libraries: A Planning and Best Practices Sourcebook by Patricia Higginbottom and Valerie Gordon
Translating Expertise: The Librarian's Role in Translational Research edited by Marisa L. Conte
Expert Searching in the Google Age by Terry Ann Jankowski
Digital Rights Management: The Librarian's Guide edited by Catherine A. Lemmer and Carla P. Wale
The Medical Library Association Guide to Data Management for Librarians edited by Lisa Federer
Developing Librarian Competencies for the Digital Age edited by Jeffrey Coghill and Roger Russell
New Methods of Teaching and Learning in Libraries by Ann Whitney Gleason
Becoming a Powerhouse Librarian: How to Get Things Done Right the First Time by Jamie Gray
Assembling the Pieces of a Systematic Review: Guide for Librarians edited by Margaret J. Foster and Sarah T. Jewell

Assembling the Pieces of a Systematic Review

Guide for Librarians

Edited by
Margaret J. Foster
Sarah T. Jewell

ROWMAN & LITTLEFIELD
Lanham • Boulder • New York • London

Published by Rowman & Littlefield
A wholly owned subsidiary of The Rowman & Littlefield Publishing Group, Inc.
4501 Forbes Boulevard, Suite 200, Lanham, Maryland 20706
www.rowman.com

Unit A, Whitacre Mews, 26-34 Stannary Street, London SE11 4AB

British Library Cataloguing in Publication Information Available

Library of Congress Cataloging-in-Publication Data Available

ISBN 9781442277014 (hardback : alk. paper) | ISBN 9781442277021 (electronic)

∞™ The paper used in this publication meets the minimum requirements of American National Standard for Information Sciences—Permanence of Paper for Printed Library Materials, ANSI/NISO Z39.48-1992.

Printed in the United States of America

Contents

Tables, Textboxes, and Figures

TABLES

TEXTBOXES

Informational

Action

Librarian's Corner

FIGURE

Preface

Systematic reviews play an important role in a variety of disciplines, including medicine, public health, and education. Across many disciplines, reviews can inform policies, change practices, and organize evidence (McKibbon 2006). Dr. Ben Goldcare, in his foreword to the book *Testing Treatments*, wrote, "The notion of systematic review—looking at the totality of evidence—is quietly one of the most important innovations in medicine over the past 30 years" (Evans, Thornton, and Chalmers 2011). The research method of systematic reviews, which uses deliberate and transparent methods to identify, critically appraise, and synthesize relevant findings, has moved to the forefront of medical research and is positioned at the top of most hierarchies of the quality of evidence (Mulrow and Cook 1998). In the education field, there have also been great strides in developing standards such as the What Works Clearinghouse initiative of the U.S. Department of Education, which uses the systematic review process as the basis for its publications (Institute of Education Sciences 2008). In fields as critical as medicine and education, where lives and futures are at stake, it is essential that the practitioners have access to the best evidence about the effectiveness of particular practices in order for them to make sound decisions.

As publications of systematic reviews have increased steadily, so has the need for authors to have the support of expert searchers. In a recent paper by Gore, there are at least a dozen citations recommending librarians in this fashion, including statements from the Cochrane Collaboration, the Campbell Collaboration, and the Institute of Medicine, now named National Academies of Sciences, Engineering, and Medicine (Gore and Jones 2015). Several medical libraries have established systematic review services, and although this has not expanded much to other disciplines yet, it is starting to be discussed.

The experiences of the librarians involved in this book can inform those looking to either launch a systematic review service or refine an existing one.

ORGANIZATION AND CONTENT

This book is organized around the steps of the review, with a few introductory chapters at the beginning to provide context for reviews and ending with chapters on how to run a systematic review service and other intersections between librarianship and systematic reviews. Each chapter is written by an expert in the field, including the editors of the book. Each step (or piece) of the review process (planning the review, identifying the studies, evaluating studies, collecting and combining data, explaining the results, and summarizing the review into a report) is covered with emphasis on information roles. The book does not go into great depth in every step, as this has been well covered by other guides and resources. However, it does provide detailed descriptions of those processes most relevant to librarianship—defining the research question and the search.

AUDIENCE AND APPLICATION

This book is intended for any librarian interested in assisting researchers in conducting reviews or conducting their own reviews, including those about to open a service to systematic review authors or those looking to improve an existing service. It has several applications: for training librarians new to systematic reviews, for those developing a new systematic review service, for those wanting to establish protocols for a current service, and as a reference for those conducting reviews or running a service.

Conducting searches for systematic reviews goes beyond expert searching and requires an understanding of the entire process of the systematic review. Just as expert searching is not fully mastered by the end of a library degree, mastering the systematic review process takes a great deal of time and practice. Attending workshops and webinars can introduce the topic, but application of the knowledge through practice is required. Running a systematic review service is complicated and requires staying informed about the latest standards, best practices, and methods.

Participating in systematic reviews is a new frontier of librarianship, in which librarians can truly become research partners with our patrons, instead of merely providing access to resources and services. This is an exciting time to be a librarian, and we welcome our readers to challenge themselves and their colleagues to expand the roles of the librarian through their active presence in this compelling new arena.

REFERENCES

Evans, I., H. Thornton, and I. Chalmers. 2011. *Testing Treatments*. London: Pinter and Martin.

Gore, G. C., and J. Jones. 2015. "Systematic Reviews and Librarians: A Primer for Managers." *Canadian Journal of Library and Information Practice and Research* 10 (1).

Institute of Education Sciences (U.S.). 2008. *What Works Clearinghouse: Procedures and Standards Handbook*. Version 2.0. Washington, DC: U.S. Department of Education, Institute of Education Sciences.

McKibbon, K. A. 2006. "Systematic Reviews and Librarians." *Library Trends* 55 (1): 202–15.

Mulrow, C. D., and D. Cook. 1998. *Systematic Reviews: Synthesis of Best Evidence for Health Care Decisions*. Philadelphia, PA: American College of Physicians.

Chapter One

Introduction to Systematic Reviews

Margaret J. Foster and Sarah T. Jewell

Most of us feel overburdened by information, although I would say the overloaded feeling comes more from coordinating all of the information and responding to it.

—David Rose

OBJECTIVES

- Describe systematic review including definitions, processes, standards, types of questions, and reasons for conducting reviews
- Detail history of systematic reviews
- List and describe international and national organizations involved in systematic reviews
- Describe role of librarians

OVERVIEW

Information overload is occurring in every discipline, with thousands of primary studies reported each year, and trying to keep up with the latest research even in a narrow field can be daunting if not impossible. There are many databases containing millions of records—over 20 million in PubMed (medicine), 1.3 million in ERIC (education), and 4 million in PsycINFO (psychology). In order to gain clarity and fully benefit from this overwhelming amount of research, knowledge syntheses are needed. The notion of syntheses is not new, with many reviews being published in an attempt to catalog, evaluate, and qualitatively or quantitatively synthesize known information. Traditional or narrative reviews have been criticized as being "haphazard, biased and subject to the idiosyncratic impressions of the individual reviewer" (Mulrow 1987). Syntheses have evolved over time, resulting in a high level of variation in approaches to reviews, which continue to develop and mature (Gough, Oliver, and Thomas 2012). The systematic review method has become the gold standard of the medical field with an estimated eleven systematic reviews publishing daily, and the method is being adopted and standardized by other disciplines (Bastian, Glasziou, and Chalmers 2010). In addition to being the method of choice for synthesis, systematic reviews are frequently the basis of guideline and policy development in many fields such as medicine, public health, and education. There are many examples which could be used to demonstrate the potential usefulness of well-done reviews. The following situation comparing two pandemics will provide insight.

A Tale of Two Pandemics

In 1918, the world was overwhelmed by a pandemic influenza designated the Spanish flu, which sickened nearly one-third of the world's population, or 500 million, and killed 50 to 100 million people, with 675,000 Americans dead (U.S. Department of Health and Human Services). As was to be expected, people were panicked. Prevention focused on lessening exposure by requiring people to wear masks, outlawing spitting on city sidewalks, and encouraging those with symptoms to avoid crowded venues such as theaters, sporting events, and church. Other preventive measures were marketed from the innocuous (onions) to a variety of elixirs (one recommended by the surgeon general), which varied in main ingredients. Consumers had no idea what would work—only the fear that they or their loved ones would be next to become ill or die.

In 2009, nearly one hundred years later, another pandemic influenza hit the world—H1N1. The Centers for Disease Control and Prevention warned the public to cover sneezes, wash hands frequently, and avoid crowded areas if symptomatic. In addition, Tamiflu (generic name: oseltamivir) was stockpiled by government agencies—the United States spent $1.3 billion while Britain spent $711 million (Associated Press 2014). Most consumers had never heard of Tamiflu but suddenly began to buy it as a precaution. Many wondered if the cost was worth it. The Cochrane Collaboration had published a systematic review prior to the outbreak in 2008 on neuraminidase inhibitors (Tamiflu is in this category) and its effectiveness for treating or preventing influenza. After the outbreak, Australian and British governments asked the Cochrane Collaboration to revisit the evidence, which was done and the authors concluded that the drug does reduce the rate of influenza-related complications such as pneumonia. Then a young physician from Japan, Keiji Hayashi, questioned the findings of the review, pointing out that it appeared that some studies appeared to be missing. Cochrane began investigating, and missing studies were eventually released by Roche, the pharmaceutical manufacturer of Tamiflu. In the latest update of the review, the authors concluded that "there were substantial problems with the design, conduct, reporting and availability of information from many of the trials" from the manufacturer and that there is insufficient evidence that Tamiflu interrupts viral transmission and reduces complications of influenza (Jefferson et al. 2014). While consumers may not have known what was effective at the time of the 2009 influenza outbreak, studies during and afterward synthesized into a well-conducted review demonstrated what was not. It is important to note that these findings have been disputed by Roche, and many governments are still buying neuraminidase inhibitors.

As demonstrated by this case study, the application of systematic reviews in medicine makes the conduct and utilization of reviews important to all. If reviews are not well done, this can lead to ineffective, inappropriate, or harmful guidelines and policies. Of course, reviews are not just published in medicine but in many disciplines and to answer a variety of question types. Chapter 2 will describe the role of systematic reviews in a variety of disciplines, how to find them, and how to evaluate them.

HISTORY OF SYSTEMATIC REVIEWS AND ORGANIZATIONS

While many of the standards for systematic reviews are coming out of medicine today, systematic reviews started around the same time in the social sciences. Glass coined the term meta-analysis in 1975, shortly thereafter publishing two articles which approached their topics in a systematic manner, one in education and one in psychotherapy. Meanwhile, Archie Cochrane published his paper called "Effectiveness and Efficiency" (1972), urging health-care providers to practice evidence-based medicine. In the late 1970s and 1980s, a group began to organize around producing systematic reviews, particularly in perinatal medicine, and then the Cochrane Centre, with funding from the British National Health Service, was formed in Oxford in October 1992. Only a year later, the group expanded its work to international areas, forming a center in Baltimore and also the Nordic Cochrane Centre. In 1994, they published the first *Cochrane Handbook*, which guides researchers in the conducting of systematic reviews, even beyond the reach of the Cochrane organization. In 1996, the Cochrane Database of Systematic Reviews was made available on the web. Today, the database includes more than 4,650 reviews and 2,015 protocols and is made freely available online, with subscriptions also available. The full Cochrane Library also includes the Database of Abstracts of Reviews of Effects, which contains quality assessments and review summaries not conducted by Cochrane; the Cochrane Central Register of Controlled Trials, an international directory of randomized controlled trials; the Cochrane Methodology Register, a bibliography of books and journal articles where researchers have reported on the methods used in randomized clinical trials; the Health Technology Assessment Database, a collection of assessment studies of medical, social, ethical, and economic implications of health-care interventions; and the NHS Economic Evaluation Database, which identifies information about the cost effectiveness of interventions. While Cochrane is known for their focus on randomized controlled trials and effectiveness reviews, they are expanding their definition of evidence-based medicine, having conducted their first qualitative reviews in 2013.

While Cochrane blazed the way for stronger evidence in medicine, Donald Campbell, an American psychologist, founded a sibling organization to Cochrane, expanding the methodology to promote systematic reviews in education, criminal justice, social policy, and social care. An exploratory meeting was held in London in 1999, including eighty-five participants from thirteen countries, and in February 2000, the Campbell Collaboration was formally established at the University of Pennsylvania.

Around the same time as the Cochrane Centre was being established, Ann Oakley set out to develop a database of evaluations of interventions in the fields of education and social welfare. In 1995, the University of London's Social Science Research Unit started a number of systematic reviews to cover fields that Cochrane was not covering, and the EPPI-Centre, the Evidence for Policy and Practice Information and Co-ordinating Centre, came into being.

ACTION BOX 1.1

Find three different types of reviews on the same topic.
Example—reviews on diabetes.
Example—reviews on educational reading interventions.
How do the reviews differ? Do they answer different types of questions? What are some of the strengths or weaknesses of the reviews?

In 1996, out of the Health Sciences Department at the University of Adelaide, South Australia, in conjunction with the Royal Adelaide Hospital, the Joanna Briggs Institute was born. The international nonprofit research and development center is focused on providing evidence-based nursing reviews,

Table 1.1. Systematic review organizations

Organization/Link	*Funding Source*	*Topics Covered*
Cochrane Collaboration, www.cochrane.org	Charity registered in England; many international centers	Effectiveness reviews; medicine
Joanna Briggs Institute, http://joannabriggs.org	International nonprofit; based in University of Adelaide, South Australia	Primarily nursing; includes qualitative reviews
Campbell Collaboration, http://www.campbellcollaboration.org	International research network	Criminal justice, education, international development, social welfare
What Works Clearinghouse, http://ies.ed.gov/ncee/wwc	Initiative of the U.S. Department of Education's National Center for Education Evaluation and Regional Assistance	Effectiveness reviews as well as primary effectiveness studies; education
International Development, http://r4d.dfid.gov.uk/SystematicReviews.aspx	UK Department for International Development	Education, health and nutrition, social sciences, environment, economic development, etc.
International Initiative for Impact Evaluation, http://www.3ieImpact.org/en/evidence/systematic-reviews	Bill & Melinda Gates Foundation, UK Department for International Development, and the William and Flora Hewlett Foundation	Effectiveness of social and economic interventions in low- and middle-income countries
Nutrition, https://ods.od.nih.gov/Research/Evidence Based_Review_Program.aspx	National Institutes of Health, Office of Dietary Supplements	Efficacy and safety of dietary supplements
Collaboration for Environmental Evidence, http://www.environmentalevidence.org	International nonprofit	Evidence synthesis on environmental policy and practice
Network for Business Sustainability, http://nbs.net/knowledge	International network of academic experts and business leaders	Systematic reviews on environmental policy, global supply chains, innovation, long-term thinking

although in recent years, it is expanding to other areas in the health sciences. Founding resource centers around the world have established this organization as a full supporter of synthesizing information to improve health and health policies. Many researchers have been trained by JBI through online courses, workshops, and conferences.

DEFINING SYSTEMATIC REVIEW

Narrative Reviews

Narrative reviews or literature reviews are the easiest term to start with when explaining systematic reviews, as they represent the type of review most students and researchers are already familiar with and have written previously. Literature reviews are usually written for one of three potential purposes—as an introduction to a primary research article, as evidence justifying the case made in a proposal, or as a general overview of a topic. When reporting primary research, literature reviews are conducted to set the context for the need of the research and to compare the findings of the author's study to previous research. In proposals for theses, dissertations, grants, and other projects, academics and practitioners need literature reviews to provide background for the prospective research. As a stand-alone product, narrative reviews organize the literature to meet a broadly defined aim, in a way that cannot be evaluated or replicated, leaving readers to wonder how to determine the value of the reviews' conclusions. Another criticism of traditional narrative reviews is that "most usually examine the results of only a small part of the research evidence, and take the claims of report authors at face value" (EPPI Centre 2015). When describing a group of studies, it is important to know the potential limitation in the collection of the studies (the risk of bias in their methods, what was lacking in their reporting, and what studies might have been missed) to determine the overall strength of the evidence. If appropriately done, "systematic reviews have been found to improve the reliability and accuracy of conclusions, clearly allying them to the scientific method" (Booth, Papaioannou, and Sutton 2012).

Systematic Reviews

Systematic reviews are research projects which are more than just an organized collection of articles; they are primary studies which provide synthesized information, built on other studies but providing new insight into a phenomenon, topic, or situation. The most straightforward and useful definition of systematic reviews, applied across all questions and disciplines is that they are reviews of the research literature using systematic and transparent methods (EPPI Centre 2015; Gough, Oliver, and Thomas 2012). These processes are the following: plan, identify, evaluate, collect and combine, explain, and summarize (PIECES) what can be ascertained from existing literature in order to answer a well-defined research question. It is the clarity of the methods that distinguishes systematic reviews from other knowledge syntheses. The logic of these methods can been applied to a wide variety of research questions, disciplines, and types of studies or evidence or literature—including determining the effectiveness of interventions, developing a theory, or assessing the implementation of policies, to name a few—so that "there can be as much variation in systematic reviews as found in primary research" (Gough, Oliver, and Thomas 2012). In trying to produce a comprehensive list of types of systematic reviews, it becomes clear that there is no consensus on terminology and that review methods are in a time of rapid development.

In their 2012 article, Gough, Thomas, and Oliver described three dimensions across which systematic reviews differ: aims and approaches; structure and components; breadth, depth, and extent of work. The aims and approach of a review can be described by the question being asked, the type of evidence the review includes, and the theoretical assumptions and ideology of the review authors. Approaches can be broadly categorized as aggregation or configuration, with most reviews utilizing both techniques. Aggregative processes focus on the homogeneity of studies (combining similar data, not necessarily quantitatively), while configurative processes determine patterns from differences in studies. The difference of these processes does not mean that reviews including quantitative studies are all aggregative and those with qualitative studies are completely configurative. The structure of a review, the number of questions it attempts to answer, and the way it maps the findings can vary widely. The scope of the review—its breadth, depth, or extent of work—differs widely as appropriate for a specific question or area of literature (Gough, Thomas, and Oliver 2012).

Specifically labeling types of systematic reviews "can lead to overgeneralizations and simplification with assumptions being made about difference between reviews that only apply to particular stages of a review or that are matters of degree rather than absolute differences" (Gough, Thomas, and Oliver 2012). Looking at the differences across these three dimensions, and how they are applied in the steps of the review, is more useful. For example, meta-analysis is one type of review, especially used by Cochrane, which focuses on randomized control trials that ask a similar question to synthesize effect size. Its difference from other reviews lies in the synthesis step. Umbrella reviews, or systematic reviews of systematic reviews, are becoming more frequent, as many topics have been summarized often. These can provide a broader picture of a topic and point out issues of quality within a particular evidence base. Their difference from other reviews lies in the fact that they seek out systematic reviews instead of primary studies.

Other Review Methods

When looking at the range of reviews from nonsystematic to systematic, there are types that lie between, such as scoping reviews and concept analyses. Scoping reviews, as described by Arksey and O'Malley in 2005 are reviews that use rigorous methods to describe the literature in a field, its volume and characteristics, to determine gaps in the literature. They differ from systematic reviews in that they do not appraise the quality of the studies and do not provide a synthesis. Concept analysis is "an activity where concepts belonging to a whole, their characteristics and relations they hold within systems of concepts are clarified and described" (Nuopponen 2010). It has been used often in fields of nursing, business, and management. More review methods will be discussed in chapters 2 and 3.

STEPS OF THE REVIEW PROCESS: PIECES

The systematic review process is not a linear process but a series of steps that are iterative. However, it is useful to think of it this way, especially for novices. There are a variety of approaches to describe the steps of reviews, varying in number and terminology of the steps. For this book, we have selected the acronym PIECES to illustrate the steps of the review: planning, identifying, evaluating, collecting and combining, explaining, and summarizing.

Planning (Chapters 2, 3, and 4)

The planning stage of the systematic review process is the most difficult, as potential authors must develop a research question that is appropriate for the systematic review method, which means they need a firm grasp of the systematic review method. Librarians can play an instructional role in this step by teaching basic systematic review methods to the researchers involved. Chapter 2 describes systematic reviews across the disciplines, where to find them and how to apply them. Chapter 3 describes conducting a reference interview in the beginning of the review to scope the research question and determine eligibility criteria. Chapter 4 describes project and data management needs for reviews, including building teams, selecting software, and setting a schedule.

Identifying (Chapters 5, 6, and 7)

This is the step that most librarians will feel the most comfortable supporting—searching potential studies to be included in the review. The most difficult part of all is translating the research question and eligibility criteria into an appropriate search strategy. Developing expert-level skills in searching is essential for this step, as well as having a great understanding of databases' content, biases, and limitations. As the search consultant for a review, it is the librarian's role to provide a well-organized, systematic, and documented search. Chapter 5 will discuss database searching; chapter 6 will highlight searching beyond databases, including grey literature; and chapter 7 will provide case studies across disciplines and question types.

Evaluating (Chapter 8)

Evaluation encompasses three processes: screening by title/abstract, selecting by reviewing the full text of study reports, and determining the risk of biases within the studies. Screening and selecting require some information management skills, which will most likely be familiar to most information specialists. Risk of bias assessment, however, may be a new area, requiring additional training. Chapter 8 will cover these processes and provide resources for further development.

Collecting and Combining Data and Explaining the Synthesis (Chapter 9)

These steps involve collecting data from each study in a systematic, objective manner and combining the studies' data with an appropriate method, then explaining the implications of the findings. Chapter 9 will describe the overall process, highlighting ways librarians could be involved. Out of all the steps described, this is most likely the one where librarians will have the least amount of engagement.

Summarizing (Chapter 10)

In the summary stage, the entire review project is pulled together to match the requirements of a journal, dissertation outline, or other report needs. However, no matter what the purpose of the report, certain information should be provided, as outlined in reporting standards such as PRISMA and others. Chapter 10 describes the various reporting standards that are available and the writing process.

WHERE DO LIBRARIANS FIT INTO THE PUZZLE OF SYSTEMATIC REVIEWS?

In reading the description of systematic reviews, most would agree that the step of identifying research is the most easily recognizable role that an information specialist could join in. Other roles include project manager, data manager, report writer, documentation of processes, or data archivist (Beverley, Booth, and Bath 2003). Librarians' role in systematic reviews has been recognized for several years, but it has only been recently recognized through some standards. For example the Institute of Medicine—now named National Academies of Sciences, Engineering, and Medicine (National Academies)—developed Standards for Systematic Reviews to be applied to "systematic reviews of the comparative effectiveness of therapeutic medical or surgical interventions" which includes two standards specifically mentioning librarians:

- Standard 3.1.1: Work with a librarian or other information specialist trained in performing systematic reviews to plan the search strategy.
- Standard 3.1.3: Use an independent librarian or other information specialist to peer review the search strategy

By naming librarians as the experts who need to be consulted, the National Academies has clearly recognized the skills of information specialists in the conduct of reviews (Eden et al. 2011).

In addition, research published in the *Journal of Clinical Epidemiology* by Rethlefsen et al. provided evidence that librarian involvement improves the quality of medical systematic reviews, particularly when they are involved to the extent of being coauthors (Rethlefsen et al. 2015). The criteria used to judge the quality of the systematic reviews were the National Academies' Recommended Standards for the Search Process and a scorecard based off of the Peer Review of Electronic Search Strategies (PRESS) (McGowan et al. 2016). Librarians have proven they are able to more effectively document the search process and make the searches reproducible, although there is still room for improvement in the quality of the searches and the reporting. While some journal editors may still question a librarian's role as a coauthor, others are rejecting papers while recommending that the authors work with a librarian to improve on the searches before resubmitting. However, librarians can become involved with even more than the search strategy development. Details on the different roles that librarians can take, aligned with each step in the PIECES process, will be provided throughout the book. In chapter 11, we map out the big picture of how to coordinate an entire systematic review service. Finally, in the concluding chapter, we will cover trends in systematic reviews and how to overcome common issues and barriers.

CONCLUSIONS

Librarians have always been collaborators in the research process, whether it be providing the resources, helping users find answers to specific questions, instructing students on how to search to discover for themselves, or as a researcher on a joint project. As a profession, librarianship continues to adapt to the evolving nature of research methods, resources, and technologies. Systematic review methods represent a growing area where librarians can and should play a vital role in collaborating on well-done research syntheses. Like a jigsaw puzzle, completed systematic reviews are greater than the pieces required to complete them. However, the pieces need to fit together well, and the processes need to be transparent and reproducible. The end product needs to be reported appropriately in order to be applied to the right situations or policies and to move the research further.

REFERENCES

Arksey, Hilary, and Lisa O'Malley. 2005. "Scoping studies: Towards a methodological framework." *International Journal of Social Research Methodology* no. 8 (1):19–32. doi: 10.1080/1364557032000119616.

Associated Press. 2014. "Study Says Billions Wasted on Tamiflu Stockpile—Which May Work No Better than Over-the-Counter Paracetemol." *National Post*, April 10. http://news.nationalpost.com/health/study-says-billions-wasted-on-stockpile-of-tamiflu-which-may-work-no-better-than-over-the-counter-paracetemol.

Bastian, Hilda, Paul Glasziou, and Iain Chalmers. 2010. "Seventy-Five Trials and Eleven Systematic Reviews a Day: How Will We Ever Keep Up?" *PLoS Med* 7 (9): e1000326. doi:10.1371/journal.pmed.1000326.

Beverley, C. A., A. Booth, and P. A. Bath. 2003. "The Role of the Information Specialist in the Systematic Review Process: A Health Information Case Study." *Health Information and Libraries Journal* 20 (2): 65–74.

Booth, Andrew, Diana Papaioannou, and Anthea Sutton. 2012. *Systematic Approaches to a Successful Literature Review*. Los Angeles: Sage. https://tamulibraries.on.worldcat.org/search?databaseList=&queryString=booth+systematic+review.

Eden, Jill, Laura Levit, Alfred Berg, and Sally Morton. 2011. *Finding What Works in Health Care*. Washington, DC: National Academies Press.

EPPI Centre. 2015. "What Is a Systematic Review?"

Gough, David, Sandy Oliver, and James Thomas. 2012. *An Introduction to Systematic Reviews*. London: Sage.

Gough, David, James Thomas, and Sandy Oliver. 2012. "Clarifying Differences between Review Designs and Methods." *Systematic Reviews* 1:28. doi:10.1186/2046-4053-1-28.

Jefferson, Tom, Mark A. Jones, Peter Doshi, Chris B. Del Mar, Rokuro Hama, Matthew J. Thompson, Elizabeth A. Spencer, et al. 2014. "Neuraminidase Inhibitors for Preventing and Treating Influenza in Adults and Children." In *Cochrane Database of Systematic Reviews*. Hoboken, NJ: Wiley.

McGowan, J., M. Sampson, D. M. Salzwedel, E. Cogo, V. Foerster, and C. Lefebvre. 2016. "PRESS Peer Review of Electronic Search Strategies: 2015 Guideline Statement." *Journal of Clinical Epidemiology* 75:40–46. doi:10.1016/j.jclinepi.2016.01.021.

Mulrow, C. D. 1987. "The Medical Review Article: State of the Science." *Annals of Internal Medicine* 106 (3): 485–88.

Nuopponen, Anita. 2010. "Methods of Concept Analysis: A Comparative Study, Part 1 of 3." *LSP Journal: Language for Special Purposes, Professional Communication, Knowledge Management, and Cognition* 1 (1): 4. http://gateway.proquest.com/openurl?ctx_ver=Z39.88-2003&xri:pqil:res_ver=0.2&res_id=xri:ilcs-us&rft_id=xri:ilcs:rec:abell:R04330425.

Rethlefsen, Melissa L., Ann M. Farrell, Leah C. Osterhaus Trzasko, and Tara J. Brigham. 2015. "Librarian Co-Authors Correlated with Higher Quality Reported Search Strategies in General Internal Medicine Systematic Reviews." *Journal of Clinical Epidemiology* 68 (6): 617–26. doi:10.1016/j.jclinepi.2014.11.025.

U.S. Department of Health and Human Services. "The Great Pandemic." Accessed July 18, 2016.

Chapter Two

The Big Picture

Finding, Evaluating, and Applying Systematic Reviews across Disciplines

Sarah Young and Erin Eldermire

Breakthrough innovation occurs when we bring down boundaries and encourage disciplines to learn from each other.

—Gyan Nagpal

OBJECTIVES

- Describe systematic reviews across disciplines
- Detail resources for locating reviews
- Describe how to evaluate systematic reviews

OVERVIEW

As a library considering a systematic review service, understanding how systematic reviews are both used and conducted in the disciplines serves as a first step toward establishing a service that meets the needs of the user community. In some fields, leading organizations similar to the Cochrane Collaboration have emerged, providing discipline-specific guidelines for systematic reviews (e.g., the Campbell Collaboration for systematic reviews in social sciences, http://www.campbellcollaboration.org). In others, methodological guidance may be lacking and the application of systematic review methodology may vary considerably in terms of rigor. These differences are due in part to variation in the types of research conducted in different disciplines. For example, research in human medicine relies heavily on well-controlled blinded experiments, such as randomized controlled trials (RCTs).

Such studies can provide high-quality, minimally biased evidence for the effectiveness of an intervention. Systematic reviews in medicine often limit included studies to RCTs and include meta-analyses that statistically combine results across studies.

Other disciplines are constrained by the limitations of study design inherent in their research environments and thus present unique methodological challenges (Petticrew 2001). For example, public health interventions are more difficult to control, and study designs such as longitudinal observational studies or retrospective cohort studies may be common. Additionally, contextualizing the results of included studies can be more challenging in public health reviews, since study populations are often diverse and heterogeneous (Petticrew 2001). In the social sciences, studies often rely on qualitative as opposed to quantitative data. These factors can make meta-analyses more difficult and can present challenges for defining inclusion and exclusion criteria for systematic reviews.

Additionally, there may be variations in the type of literature consulted, including different optimal approaches to identifying grey literature. The librarian can play an important role in identifying subject-specific databases and information resources depending on the research question and discipline area. Grey literature may take on different shapes in different areas of research. For example, while unpublished clinical trials are important to reviews in medicine, cooperative extension reports and documents may critically inform a research question in agricultural science.

Given these disciplinary variations, as well as the fact that broadly accepted and vetted systematic review guidelines may not be available for a field, the support of researchers doing systematic reviews can be particularly challenging to the librarian. There are several approaches librarians can take to learn about how systematic reviews are applied in a field. Exploring published systematic reviews in high-quality journals can be helpful. Searching journal author guidelines for standards or requirements for systematic review submissions may also be illuminating. Additionally, searching for existing guidance documents or evidence-producing organizations in a field may be fruitful. Table 2.1 provides several resources for methodological guidance in a number of disciplines in which advances in adapting systematic review methodology have been made.

The following sections provide some examples of how systematic reviews are applied across a number of fields. A brief context for systematic reviews in the field, examples of topics addressed, and resources for methodological guidance are provided. The fields covered below include medicine, education, software engineering, environmental science and ecology, and agriculture and veterinary medicine. These are fields in which systematic reviews

Table 2.1. Guidance and resources for conducting systematic reviews by discipline

Resource	*URL*	*Discipline/subject areas covered*
Campbell Collaboration Resource Center	http://www.campbellcollaboration.org/resources/resource_center.php	Crime and justice, education, international development, social welfare
Cochrane Handbook for Systematic Reviews of Interventions	http://handbook.cochrane.org	Healthcare, clinical medicine, health services
Cochrane Handbook for Diagnostic Test Accuracy Reviews (in development)	http://dta.cochrane.org/handbook-dta-reviews	Medical diagnostic research
EPPI-Centre Methods for Conducting Systematic Reviews	http://eppi.ioe.ac.uk/cms/LinkClick.aspx?fileticket=hQBu8y4uVwI%3D	Education, social policy, health promotion, economic development, crime, other social sciences
Guidelines for Performing Systematic Literature Reviews in Software Engineering	http://community.dur.ac.uk/ebse/guidelines.php	Software engineering
Guidelines for Systematic Reviews in Environmental Management	http://www.environmentalevidence.org/information-for-authors	Environmental science, conservation biology
Guidelines for Systematic Reviews of Health Promotion and Public Health	http://ph.cochrane.org/sites/ph.cochrane.org/files/uploads/HPPH_systematic_review_handbook.pdf	Public health
National Academies	http://iom.nationalacademies.org/Reports/2011/Finding-What-Works-in-Health-Care-Standards-for-Systematic-Reviews/Standards.aspx	Comparative effectiveness research of therapeutic medical and surgical interventions
Methods Guide for Effectiveness and Comparative Effectiveness Reviews	http://effectivehealthcare.ahrq.gov/index.cfm/search-for-guides-reviews-and-reports/?pageaction=displayproduct&productid=318	Effectiveness, comparative effectiveness, and comparative harms of health-care interventions
Systematic Reviews in the Social Sciences: A Practical Guide, by Mark Petticrew and Helen Roberts	http://www.wiley.com/WileyCDA/WileyTitle/productCd-1405121106.html	Social sciences including psychology, education, urban policy, and other areas

are conducted, but by no means are systematic reviews limited to these disciplines.

Medicine

In medicine, systematic reviews are largely used to inform practice, specifically in creating clinical practice guidelines, which are recommendations meant to guide patient care by providing evidence and comparing benefits and harms of alternative treatments. The National Academies has implemented practice guidelines after gathering multidisciplinary experts to run systematic reviews (http://www.nhlbi.nih.gov/health-pro/guidelines/about). In nursing, the Joanna Briggs Institute is an entity that focuses on evidence transfer and implementation of systematic reviews (http://joannabriggs.org/jbi-approach.html). The Cochrane Collaboration leads the way in providing standards for medical systematic reviews. While they largely focus on reviews of randomized controlled trials, they are expanding their reach to include qualitative studies as well, publishing an approach known as Confidence in the Evidence from Reviews of Qualitative Research (CERQual; http://journals.plos.org/plosmedicine/article?id=10.1371/journal.pmed.1001895). Cochrane recognizes that reports on the effectiveness of interventions is not sufficient evidence for informing policy decisions, and CERQual is designed to guide the synthesis of qualitative reviews that address the feasibility and acceptability of potential health-care solutions.

Education

The importance of evidence synthesis in education was established in the 1970s with the work of Gene Glass who coined the term meta-analysis. He noted, "In education research, we need more scholarly effort concentrated on the problem of finding the knowledge that lies untapped in completed research studies" (Glass 1976). The field of education embraced systematic reviews early on and has pushed to advance the application of systematic review methods to educational research (Davies 2000; Evans and Benefield 2001; Hargreaves 1996). Systematic reviews in education cover a wide range of topics, including teaching and learning methods, optimizing the classroom environment, and assessing achievement measures (Davies 2000). In addition, Borrego emphasized the utility of systematic reviews for stimulating innovation and identifying new areas of study in engineering education (Borrego, Foster, and Froyd 2014).

For guidance in conducting systematic reviews of education research, the Campbell Collaboration and the EPPI-Centre (Evidence for Policy and Practice Information and Co-ordinating Centre) are helpful resources. The

EPPI-Centre's Methods References page (http://eppi.ioe.ac.uk/cms/Default.aspx?tabid=1919) provides a bibliography of guidance documents for conducting reviews in education and other social science fields. Both Campbell and the EPPI-Centre can be good sources of high-quality examples of systematic reviews in education. Additionally, *Systematic Reviews in the Social Sciences: A Practical Guide*, by Petticrew and Roberts, is a useful resource for conducting reviews in education and other social science fields (Petticrew and Roberts 2006).

Software Engineering

The idea of evidence-based software engineering was first proposed in 2004 (Kitchenham, Dyb, and Jorgensen 2004). Based on the model of evidence-based medicine, Kitchenham et al. suggested that decision making in areas such as technology adoption and software development practices would benefit from drawing on research evidence, rather than relying on expert opinion or being swayed by market and management pressures (Kitchenham, Dyb, and Jorgensen 2004). Examples of systematic review topics in software engineering include the optimization of virtual keyboards and software cost-estimation strategies (Gomide et al. 2015; Jorgensen and Shepperd 2007).

A Compendex search of "systematic reviews and software engineering" will reveal a wide array of literature on this topic. However, the quality of systematic reviews in this field varies widely, and clear standards are lacking (Da Silva et al., 2011). A set of guidelines was developed by a group affiliated with Keele University and the University of Durham in the United Kingdom. These guidelines, last updated in 2007, are available on the Evidence-Based Software Engineering website (http://community.dur.ac.uk/ebse), which also provides examples of software engineering systematic reviews and systematic review protocols. Guidelines and recommendations continue to evolve in this field, and several authors have critically evaluated the application of the methodology, emphasizing the need for more research, training, and methodological support (Babar and Zhang 2009; Kitchenham and Brereton 2013).

Environmental Science and Ecology

Systematic reviews are increasingly conducted in the fields of environmental science and ecology. They can be particularly useful to inform environmental policy making, providing unbiased scientific guidance to policy development (Bilotta, Milner, and Boyd 2014). In regard to ecology, Lortie (2014) noted that meta-analyses, as a form of evidence synthesis, are increasingly common, yet systematic reviews remain relatively rare. He emphasized the role of systematic reviews in identifying research gaps in ecology. In addition to meta-analyses and systematic reviews, "evidence mapping," or systematic mapping, has gained some traction in these and related fields (Dicks, Walsh, and Sutherland 2014). Evidence mapping is an evidence synthesis approach in which evidence-oriented studies such as systematic reviews, meta-analyses, and impact evaluations are systematically gathered and visually distilled to demonstrate research gaps and saturation points (McKinnon et al. 2015). As with systematic reviews, evidence maps require expertise in searching scholarly and grey literature and could present other new opportunities for engaging in scholarly research.

The Collaboration for Environmental Evidence (CEE; http://www.environmentalevidence.org) is a leading international organization for the support of systematic reviews in environmental science and conservation biology. They have produced systematic reviews since 2004 and maintain published guidelines for conducting systematic reviews in environmental management. Conservation Evidence (http://www.conservationevidence.com), based at the University of Cambridge, is another organization with a focus on evidence-based decision making for biological conservation. Conservation Evidence extracts information from major conservation journals, specialist journals, and grey literature and makes available relevant reviews from the CEE.

Agriculture and Veterinary Medicine

A nascent movement of evidence-based agriculture is underway, presenting an opportunity for agricultural librarians and land grant institutions to engage in new ways with faculty research (Fisher 2014). As more and more agricultural research and data become available, the need to synthesize this research grows. Topics such as tillage practices and water quality are examples of areas that might benefit from systematic reviews. For guidance on conducting systematic reviews in agriculture, one can draw from the previously mentioned environmental evidence organizations. The Collaboration for Environmental Evidence and Conservation Evidence, mentioned in the previous section, both address topics in agricultural science.

As for veterinary medicine, systematic reviews are becoming more common in this field as well, with research on both companion and livestock animals. Sargeant and O'Connor published a series of articles discussing systematic reviews in animal agriculture and veterinary medicine and provided discipline-specific methodological guidance. They note several challenges to synthesizing evidence in these fields including the scarcity of randomized controlled trials, the challenges of drawing conclusions across studies on different species, and the importance of factoring in considerations beyond efficacy including economic, food safety, and animal welfare issues (Sargeant and O'Connor 2014).

FINDING SYSTEMATIC REVIEWS

Finding systematic reviews can present unique challenges and is yet another way in which librarians can support users. Scholars and health-care practitioners alike may look for systematic reviews for any number of reasons. In addition to the examples highlighted earlier in this chapter, another common reason to look for systematic reviews is to prepare for conducting one's own systematic review. Before embarking on the task of conducting a systematic review, potential authors check the literature to ensure that one that addresses the question at hand is not in process or has not been published previously. When planning a systematic review, individuals can search the published literature and systematic review registries for this reason, as well as to help identify the bodies of research that could benefit from a systematic review.

In addition, authors may be preparing to update an existing systematic review. While it is recommended that Cochrane reviews are updated about every two years, recommendations for updating systematic reviews in other disciplines are still debated (Higgins, Green, and Cochrane Collaboration 2008). Shojania found that the time frame in which systematic reviews require updating varied from over ten years after publication to before a completed systematic review had even been published (Shojania et al. 2007).

Once researchers have concluded that no systematic reviews have already been conducted on their research question, they may look for systematic reviews on related topics to help define their question and inform inclusion/exclusion criteria. Just as authors of literature reviews use the existing literature to build an understanding of their inquiries, authors of systematic reviews can also draw on the literature, including related systematic reviews. An important component of systematic reviews is the search strategy used to retrieve literature, and related reviews can be a great tool for helping the authors build their own complete search strategy. Reviews that include searches on the same topic can be particularly useful: since many systematic reviews include the name of the databases that were searched and the search strategies used for each database, authors can refer to those well-defined protocols to help build their own, comprehensive search.

Finally, systematic reviews can be an excellent source of research articles and studies for potential inclusion in an ongoing review. Systematic reviewers go to great lengths to identify studies that meet their criteria, including hand searching print journals and conference proceedings and contacting researchers in the field who may know of ongoing studies firsthand. Thus, systematic reviews on related topics may have identified studies that would not appear in database searches. Checking the references of systematic reviews can help ensure that possibly relevant studies are not missed.

TEXTBOX 2.1. REASONS FOR SEEKING SYSTEMATIC REVIEWS

Knowledge and decision making

- Identifying knowledge gaps in research and new areas for inquiry
- Finding evidence to inform decision making in practice and policy development

Preparing for a systematic review

- Avoiding duplication of efforts in preparing for a systematic review
- Informing research question development and inclusion/exclusion criteria for a systematic review
- Search term harvesting for search strategy development and guidance for database and grey literature searching for a systematic review
- Identifying existing studies for inclusion in a review that may not have been found in database searches
- Updating a systematic review

Where to Look for Systematic Reviews

As the utilization of systematic reviews increases, databases and repositories that index and store systematic reviews will no doubt proliferate. While it is impractical to provide recommendations for all the resources that can be helpful when looking for systematic reviews, we provide some guidance below. The motivation for seeking out systematic reviews will also shape the approach used in searching for them. For instance, a clinician or policy maker who is looking for evidence may search a bibliographic database such as PubMed or PsycINFO, while a researcher conducting a systematic review will search in additional places, such as systematic review protocol repositories.

Protocol Registries

For those embarking on a systematic review, an early step in the process is to develop a protocol in which the investigators clearly define the objectives, parameters, and search strategies to be used throughout the process. Once the protocol is developed, it can be registered. Registration helps to minimize duplication of effort and promotes transparency in the systematic review process by providing a permanent record of prospective reviews (Shamseer et al. 2015).

A prominent protocol registry is PROSPERO (http://www.crd.york.ac.uk/PROSPERO), an internationally supported organization that maintains a database of prospectively registered systematic reviews in health and social care. The Cochrane and Campbell Collaborations publish protocols for prospective reviews in their respective fields, as does the Agency for Healthcare Research and Quality.

Those who search a systematic review protocol registry can expect to find protocols with registry numbers and basic information (e.g., prospective title, anticipated/actual start date, anticipated completion date, stage of review upon registration, contact information, organizational affiliation, funding, conflicts of interest), as well as methodological information (e.g., review question(s), searches, domains, populations, interventions, controls, study types to be included, context, outcomes, risk of bias, data synthesis strategy) (Centre for Reviews and Dissemination 2016).

Systematic Review Producers

As discussed previously, organizations have been established that specifically operate to produce systematic reviews and provide guidance for conducting systematic reviews. Thus, their websites can be good places to start in a search for systematic reviews. The Cochrane Database of Systematic Reviews (http://www.cochrane.org) is the premiere resource for systematic reviews in health and human medicine, particularly for reviews registered with the Cochrane Collaboration. Likewise, the Campbell Library of Systematic Reviews (http://www.campbellcollaboration.org/lib) hosts reviews that focus on social issues, education, and international development, even those published elsewhere. In addition to Campbell and Cochrane, there are a number of other organizations that carry out systematic reviews and generate evidence-oriented studies. The Joanna Briggs Institute (http://www.joannabriggs.org/research/registered_titles.aspx), an organization that supports the improvement of global health care, hosts a systematic review registry as well.

Bibliographic Databases

Bibliographic databases can be useful when looking for systematic reviews. For medical systematic reviews, medical databases are a natural place to start. Embase (https://www.elsevier.com/embase) and PubMed (http://www.ncbi.nlm.nih.gov/pubmed) both index a wealth of systematic reviews and provide filters that can help to quickly narrow results to only systematic reviews after an initial search.

Web of Science (http://wokinfo.com) and Scopus (https://www.elsevier.com/solutions/scopus) are especially useful when searching for systematic reviews that fall outside of the medical realm. These two databases index across numerous disciplines that have begun to utilize the systematic review methodology more recently.

Many standards for systematic reviews call for the term *systematic review* to be used in the title of the paper. In all of the bibliographic databases mentioned here, as well as many others, a simple yet effective strategy for finding systematic reviews is to incorporate a title search for the term *systematic review*. Although not all systematic reviews include this term in the title, this standard is relatively widely accepted.

Other Systematic Review Databases

In addition to the resources listed above, there are many databases specifically designed to facilitate the discovery of systematic reviews and other evidence-oriented studies. The Trip Database (https://www.tripdatabase.com) is a free search engine that focuses on supporting evidence-based medicine and includes systematic reviews. The Systematic Review Data Repository (http://srdr.ahrq.gov) is a relatively new open and searchable archive of systematic reviews, including the data products of systematic reviews, such as extraction forms (Ip et al. 2012). Discipline-specific databases for systematic reviews are also available, although to date, most of them center around health care and medicine. Table 2.2 provides a list of some examples of such databases.

EVALUATING SYSTEMATIC REVIEWS

As systematic reviews are published across different disciplines and fields and in different journals, a variety of standards are used for conducting and reporting. Despite this variety, it is important to evaluate the reviews with a critical eye on the methods used (Shea et al. 2007). Although the methods and rigor of systematic review processes vary, the principles by which systematic reviews are evaluated are similar. Two major ways by which systematic reviews in any discipline can be evaluated are transparency and appropriate methods.

If a systematic review's methods are not transparent, it cannot be evaluated and its validity cannot be determined. Systematic reviews that are well reported and reproducibly transparent can be accurately updated and can

Table 2.2. Databases of reviews in specific disciplines

Databases/link	*Discipline*
3ie, http://www.3ieimpact.org/evidence/systematic-reviews	Social and economic interventions in low- and middle-income countries
American Dental Association, Center for Evidence-Based Dentistry, http://ebd.ada.org/en/evidence/evidence-by-topic	Dentistry reviews
DoPHER, http://eppi.ioe.ac.uk/webdatabases4/Intro.aspx?ID=9	Health promotion and public health effectiveness reviews
Network Business Sustainability Reviews, http://nbs.net/knowledge	Business reviews
psycBITE, http://www.psycbite.com	Treatments for psychological problems and consequence of acquired brain impairment
PEDro, http://www.pedro.org.au	Physiotherapy
SpeechBITE, http://speechbite.com	Speech pathology treatment

facilitate subsequent systematic reviews to fill exposed knowledge gaps (Higgins, Green, and Cochrane Collaboration 2008). Several factors can contribute to whether a systematic review is reproducible, including, but not limited to, whether the literature search that was conducted was fully documented, appropriate databases were used to search for information, documented inclusion/exclusion criteria were used, and data syntheses were carried out in a statistically sound manner.

The methods of the review also need to be appropriate, not just reported well. The question needs to be appropriate for the systematic review method, the eligibility criteria for included studies need to be set correctly, and the search for relevant literature should be comprehensive to minimize any risk that relevant studies may be omitted from consideration (Abalos et al. 2001). The processes for appraising and coding the studies should follow standards and validated methods (discussed in chapters 8 and 9) to ensure that the evidence is presented and placed in proper context.

Critical Appraisal Tools

Soon after systematic review methods began to be applied to fields beyond human medicine, researchers began to publish methods by which to appraise the validity and applicability of systematic reviews. In 1994, Oxman, Cook, and Guyatt published a *User's Guide to the Medical Literature: How to Use an Overview*, in which they propose key questions to ask when evaluating systematic reviews to be used for clinical decisions (Oxman, Cook, and Guyatt 1994). Abalos built on this to provide clear guidelines for evaluating clinically focused systematic reviews (Abalos et al. 2001). To assess medical and nonmedical systematic reviews, the guidelines of the Joanna Briggs Institute for Evidence Based Nursing and Midwifery can be widely applied (Evans and Chang 2000).

Following these publications, a number of tools have been developed to assist in the critical appraisal of systematic reviews, the most notable of which is AMSTAR (Zeng et al. 2015). AMSTAR (A MeaSurement Tool to Assess systematic Reviews, http://amstar.ca) is a simple checklist that takes only a few minutes to complete. AMSTAR was methodologically developed, tested, and vetted by experts and has stood up to retests validating its utility (Shea, Bouter, et al. 2007; Shea, Grimshaw, et al. 2007; Shea et al. 2009). This web-based tool (with a printable version) poses simple questions with minimum guidelines for each dimension of a systematic review and provides a score to help illustrate whether the systematic review meets those standards.

Another web-based tool was developed by Whiting et al. and named ROBIS (risk of bias in systematic reviews), which was designed to determine the risk of bias within the systematic reviews of medically related reviews in areas of intervention effectiveness, etiology, diagnosis, and prognosis (Whiting et al. 2016). The assessment addressed potential concerns for reviews' eligibility criteria, methods to identify studies, data collection, study appraisal, appropriate synthesis, and interpretation.

Other useful systematic review appraisal tools include a worksheet produced by CEBM (Centre for Evidence Based Medicine; http://www.cebm.net/critical-appraisal), a critical appraisal worksheet for systematic reviews, and the SURE critical appraisal worksheet by Cardiff University (http://www.cardiff.ac.uk/insrv/libraries/sure/checklists.html). CASP (Critical Appraisal Skills Programme; http://www.casp-uk.net/), an organization that aims to provide (Shea et al. 2007) tools for anybody using research evidence to guide their decision making, has developed several checklists, including one for systematic reviews. There are too many critical appraisal tools to list

Table 2.3. Selected systematic review critical appraisal tools

Resource	*URL*
AMSTAR (A MeaSurement Tool to Assess systematic Reviews)	http://amstar.ca
CASP (Critical Appraisal Skills Programme)	http://www.casp-uk.net
ROBIS (risk of bias in systematic reviews)	robis-tool.info
SIGN (Scottish Intercollegiate Guidelines Network)	http://www.sign.ac.uk

here, including many useful "mashup" versions. Researchers are steadily working to improve these tools, and others will no doubt be developed and refined in the future.

> **ACTION BOX 2.1**
>
> Find a systematic review or two on a topic in your discipline of choice. Use AMSTAR guidelines to evaluate the review. If comparing two reviews, which one seems the stronger evidence overall? Are there things you would have done differently if you were conducting the review? Start imagining yourself in the shoes of the researcher, rather than just the reader.

APPLICATIONS OF SYSTEMATIC REVIEWS TO PRACTICE AND POLICY MAKING

It is well established that systematic reviews can be an effective way of synthesizing and distilling large numbers of publications to draw conclusions about what is or is not known about a particular intervention or treatment. But how do systematic reviews get used in practice? How do systematic reviews translate to decision making and policy changes? The process of translation and implementation is well beyond the scope of this book. However, understanding the context in which a systematic review will be interpreted is critical to both developing meaningful research questions and providing actionable findings.

The anticipated audience for a systematic review should be considered. The audience may vary depending on the discipline and purpose of the review. Systematic reviews in medicine will likely be referenced by clinicians in making decisions for patient care. Reviews in public health may impact practices and programming decisions by community organizations and public health practitioners, but they could also have implications at the public policy level. Systematic reviews additionally serve to identify existing knowledge gaps and may be used by academic researchers to identify new and urgent avenues of inquiry. Thus, considering the audience in the final write-up of a systematic review is critical to effectively communicating the meaning and implications of a review's findings.

Implications for Library Services

The wide application of systematic review methodology has implications for how and why a library may decide to develop a formal service. Systematic reviews and other types of evidence synthesis play an increasingly important role for researchers and practitioners alike. Thus, thinking broadly about how systematic reviews are used in different disciplines can help libraries shape their service appropriately, as well as leverage opportunities to uniquely engage with user communities.

In addition to systematic reviews, other types of reviews applying a systematic method may be employed. Rapid reviews, for example, use a systematic approach to provide guidance quickly and address emerging issues in a field, allowing program leaders and policy makers to make evidence-based decisions. Academic libraries that work frequently with researchers engaged with community practitioners, or that work with the practitioners directly, may find that the rapid review approach is a better-suited methodology to inform their user community's evidence-based practice.

Systematic reviews can be used to support grant-seeking activity. Today, a greater competition for a smaller pot of funding requires more novel innovations aimed at filling identifiable research gaps. Systematic reviews can serve to identify such knowledge gaps. At the same time, they require little funding themselves (albeit considerable time and effort) and can make potentially important contributions to a field.

It is important to note that systematic review services and support are not necessarily restricted to faculty and advanced researchers. Graduate students may conduct systematic reviews as part of their theses or dissertations or may be involved in systematic reviews with their faculty advisors. In addition, the methodology used to search for literature in a systematic review can benefit the process of writing a traditional narrative review. Applying a systematic method can result in a more comprehensive review that is less biased and more transparent than a traditional literature review. In this way, a well-researched dissertation literature review can stand alone as a publishable contribution to the field.

REFERENCES

Abalos, E., G. Carroli, M. E. Mackey, and E. Bergel. 2001. "Critical Appraisal of Systematic Reviews." The WHO Reproductive Health Library. Geneva: World Health Organization. http://www.who.int/entity/rhl/Critical%20appraisal%20of%20systematic%20reviews.pdf.

Babar, M.A., and He Zhang. 2009. "Systematic Literature Reviews in Software Engineering: Preliminary Results from Interviews with Researchers." In *3rd International Symposium on Empirical Software Engineering and Measurement, 2009. ESEM 2009*, 346–55.

Bilotta, G. S., A. M. Milner, and I. Boyd. 2014. "On the Use of Systematic Reviews to Inform Environmental Policies." *Environmental Science and Policy* 42: 67–77.

Borrego, M., M. J. Foster, and J. E. Froyd. 2014. "Systematic Literature Reviews in Engineering Education and Other Developing Interdisciplinary Fields." *Journal of Engineering Education* 103 (1): 45–76.

Centre for Reviews and Dissemination. "PROSPERO—International Prospective Register of Systematic Reviews." PROSPERO, November 4, 2015. http://www.crd.york.ac.uk/PROSPERO.

Da Silva, F. Q. B., A. L. M. Santos, S. Soares, A. C. C. Frana, C. V. F. Monteiro, and F. F. MacIel. 2011. "Six Years of Systematic Literature Reviews in Software Engineering: An Updated Tertiary Study." *Information and Software Technology* 53 (9): 899–913.

Davies, P. 2000. "The Relevance of Systematic Reviews to Educational Policy and Practice." *Oxford Review of Education* 26 (3–4): 364–78.

Dicks, L. V., J. C. Walsh, and W. J. Sutherland. 2014. "Organising Evidence for Environmental Management Decisions: A '4S' Hierarchy." *Trends in Ecology and Evolution* 29 (11): 607–13.

Evans, David, and Anne Chang. 2000. "Appraising Systematic Reviews." Changing Practice: Evidence Based Practice Information Sheets for Health Professionals. http://www.joannabriggs.edu.au/CP1.pdf.

Evans, J., and P. Benefield. 2001. "Systematic Reviews of Educational Research: Does the Medical Model Fit?" *British Educational Research Journal* 27 (5): 527–41.

Fisher, Madeline. 2014. "Making the Case for Evidence-Based Agriculture." *CSA News* 59 (5): 4.

Glass, Gene V. 1976. "Primary, Secondary, and Meta-Analysis of Research." *Educational Researcher* 5 (10): 3–8.

Gomide, R. S., L. F. B. Loja, E. L. Flores, R. P. Lemos, S. D. Carvalho, and R. E. M. Silva. 2015. "A Systematic Review on Methods and Techniques for Optimizing Assistive Virtual Keyboards." *IEEE Latin America Transactions* 13 (8): 2687–93.

Hargreaves, David H. 1996. "Teaching as a Research-Based Profession: Possibilities and Prospects." Presented at the Teacher Training Agency Annual Lecture, University of Cambridge, 1996. http://eppi.ioe.ac.uk/cms/Portals/0/PDF%20reviews%20and%20summaries/TTA%20Hargreaves%20lecture.pdf.

Higgins, Julian P. T., Sally Green, and Cochrane Collaboration. 2008. *Cochrane Handbook for Systematic Reviews of Interventions*. Chichester, England; Hoboken, NJ: Wiley-Blackwell.

Ip, S., N. Hadar, S. Keefe, C. Parkin, R. Iovin, E. M. Balk, and J. Lau. 2012. "A Web-Based Archive of Systematic Review Data." *Systematic Reviews* 1 (1).

Jorgensen, M., and M. Shepperd. 2007. "A Systematic Review of Software Development Cost Estimation Studies." *IEEE Transactions on Software Engineering* 33 (1): 33–53.

Kitchenham, B. A., T. Dyb, and M. Jorgensen. 2004. "Evidence-Based Software Engineering." In *Proceedings of the 26th International Conference on Software Engineering*, 273–81. ICSE '04. Washington, DC: IEEE Computer Society.

Kitchenham, B., and P. Brereton. 2013. "A Systematic Review of Systematic Review Process Research in Software Engineering." *Information and Software Technology* 55 (12): 2049–75.

Lortie, C. J. 2014. Formalized synthesis opportunities for ecology: Systematic reviews and meta-analyses. Oikos, 123(8), 897–902. https://doi.org/10.1111/j.1600-0706.2013.00970.x

McKinnon, M. C., S. H. Cheng, R. Garside, Y. J. Masuda, and D. C. Miller. 2015. "Sustainability: Map the Evidence." *Nature* 528 (7581): 185–87.

Oxman, A. D., D. J. Cook, and G. H. Guyatt. 1994. "Users' Guides to the Medical Literature. VI. How to Use an Overview. Evidence-Based Medicine Working Group." *JAMA* 272 (17): 1367–71.

Petticrew, M. 2001. "Systematic Reviews from Astronomy to Zoology: Myths and Misconceptions." *BMJ (Clinical Research Ed.)* 322 (7278): 98–101.

Petticrew, Mark, and Helen Roberts. 2006. *Systematic Reviews in the Social Sciences: A Practical Guide*. Malden, MA: Oxford: Blackwell Publishers.

Sargeant, J. M., and A. M. O'Connor. 2014. "'One-Stop Shopping' for Information on Conducting Systematic Reviews and Meta-Analysis in Animal Agriculture and Veterinary Medicine." *Zoonoses and Public Health* 61 Suppl 1: 2.

Shamseer, L., D. Moher, M. Clarke, D. Ghersi, A. Liberati, M. Petticrew, P. Shekelle, L. A. Stewart, and PRISMA-P Group. 2015. "Preferred Reporting Items for Systematic Review and Meta-Analysis Protocols (PRISMA-P) 2015: Elaboration and Explanation." *BMJ (Clinical Research Ed.)* 349:g7647.

Shea, Beverley J., Lex M. Bouter, Joan Peterson, Maarten Boers, Neil Andersson, Zulma Ortiz, Tim Ramsay, Annie Bai, Vijay K. Shukla, and Jeremy M. Grimshaw. 2007. "External Validation of a Measurement Tool to Assess Systematic Reviews (AMSTAR)." *PLoS ONE* 2, (12): e1350.

Shea, B. J., J. M. Grimshaw, G. A. Wells, M. Boers, N. Andersson, C. Hamel, A. C. Porter, P. Tugwell, D. Moher, and L. M. Bouter. 2007. "Development of AMSTAR: A Measurement Tool to Assess the Methodological Quality of Systematic Reviews." *BMC Medical Research Methodology* 7:10.

Shea, Beverley J., Candyce Hamel, George A. Wells, Lex M. Bouter, Elizabeth Kristjansson, Jeremy Grimshaw, David A. Henry, and Maarten Boers. 2009. "AMSTAR Is a Reliable and Valid Measurement Tool to Assess the Methodological Quality of Systematic Reviews." *Journal of Clinical Epidemiology* 62 (10): 1013–20.

Shojania, K. G., M. Sampson, M. T. Ansari, J. Ji, S. Doucette, and D. Moher. 2007. "How Quickly Do Systematic Reviews Go Out of Date? A Survival Analysis." *Annals of Internal Medicine* 147 (4): 224–33.

Whiting, Penny, Jelena Savović, Julian P. T. Higgins, Deborah M. Caldwell, Barnaby C. Reeves, Beverley Shea, Philippa Davies, Jos Kleijnen, and Rachel Churchill.

2016. "ROBIS: A New Tool to Assess Risk of Bias in Systematic Reviews Was Developed." *Journal of Clinical Epidemiology* 69: 225–34. doi:10.1016/j.jclinepi.2015.06.005.

Zeng, X., Y. Zhang, J. S. Kwong, C. Zhang, S. Li, F. Sun, Y. Niu, and L. Du. 2015. "The Methodological Quality Assessment Tools for Preclinical and Clinical Studies, Systematic Review and Meta-Analysis, and Clinical Practice Guideline: A Systematic Review." *Journal of Evidence-Based Medicine* 8 (1): 2–10.

Chapter Three

Planning the Review, Part 1

The Reference Interview

Julie H. Schiavo and Margaret J. Foster

The famous dictum, "Speech was given to man to conceal thought," is often forcibly brought to mind by the ingenuity with which visitors to the reference-room succeed in hiding their desires behind their questions. And right here lies the opportunity for the exercise of one of the greatest gifts of the successful librarian—the ability by skillful [sic] questioning, without appearance of curiosity or impertinence, to extract from the vaguest, most general requests, a clear idea of what the inquirer really needs.

—Eleanor B. Woodruff, 1897

OBJECTIVES

- Detail the needs during the planning stage
- Describe the reference interview for the initial meeting
- Describe determining the feasibility of research question to match the systematic review method

OVERVIEW

Systematic reviews, as with any other request for assistance posed to librarians, must begin with a mutual understanding between the librarian and client. Ms. Woodruff's statement still holds true today: librarians must use their communication and critical thinking skills to comprehend the true meaning and purpose of clients' requests. The initial reference interview for a systematic review project will follow many of the traditional techniques employed by librarians in any library. There are many philosophies regarding the proper approach and most effective techniques used in a reference interview. Although these philosophies have evolved over time and are often situation specific, the main goal remains the same: to clarify and understand the research question before moving into searching (Kern, Woodward, and Woodward 2011).

INITIAL MEETING

The reference interview is the first step for the librarian to be successful in consulting and collaborating in the systematic review process. During this meeting, the researchers and the librarian must define the scope of the review, establish clear expectations of the project, and develop a rapport of mutual respect (Bates 1998).

Research has shown that if clients have a positive interaction with librarians rather than simply receiving the best information, they are more willing to return. The key to providing this positive interaction is by actively listening to the client (Durrance 1995). The Guidelines for Behavioral Performance of Reference and Information Service Providers, developed by the Reference and User Services Association (a division of the American Library Association), provides a list of actions to follow during a reference interview to provide clients with high-level customer service. Active listening techniques include giving the client complete attention, paraphrasing the client's question, asking for clarification when necessary, and providing constructive feedback (Bates 1998; Kern, Woodward, and Woodward 2011). Part of active listening includes selecting the appropriate type of questions at the right time: open or closed.

Most information garnered through the interview process will be obtained with open questions. Open questions will encourage the client and elucidate the information need using their own terms. There is no fixed response to an open question; yes or no will not be a sufficient response. If a topic is unfamiliar to the librarian, open questions will provide explanations and insights on the subject. Closed questions should be used strategically to avoid leading the client down an unintended path or limiting options prematurely. They present the user with a limited number of responses and focus narrowly on one particular subject. Once there is a mutual understanding of the client's information needs, closed questions will provide the necessary details to craft an extensive search strategy and provide the types of results sought by the client (Kern, Woodward, and Woodward 2011). Table 3.1 lists example questions as open or closed that one might consider during a reference interview for reviews.

Table 3.1. Closed versus open questions

Closed question	*Open question*
Are you following a specific protocol for this systematic review?	Why do you want to conduct this review?
Have you done any searches on your own?	What kinds of results have you found with your own searches?
Do you have articles which you have already found that you want to include?	How much information are you expecting? (How many studies are you expecting to include in the systematic review?)
Are there any related systematic reviews to your topic? Are there any studies that you know should be included in this review?	Have you found any other systematic reviews on this topic?
Is this particular term appropriate for this search?	What other terms should be included in the search?

A systematic review project requires the client and librarian to be clear on several aspects of the project beyond the traditional reference interview questions. During the initial meeting, several questions need to be answered, as detailed in box 3.1. If both the researcher and the librarian are on the same page and understand the requirements, expectations, and intents of the systematic review, it will be far less likely that research will have to be altered or repeated, saving large amounts of time and effort (Bates 1998). A clear decision by the librarian or his or her manager should be made as to what level of service will be provided, based on time and resources. If time does not permit a librarian to have full involvement in a systematic review, for example, perhaps an advisory role could be offered. More details about the role of the librarian in the review process will be provided in chapter 11 including models of consultation and developing a systematic review service.

Agreeing on the Definition of Systematic Review

Often, a client will request help in doing a systematic review with little understanding of what a systematic review entails. As discussed in chapter 1, the definition of systematic reviews can be problematic, especially in disciplines which have only begun to explore the method and provide few if any standards to researchers and practitioners in the field. In the initial meeting, discussing the ways systematic reviews differ from traditional reviews is a good starting point. Also, providing the client with relevant systematic reviews compared to their topic, as discussed in the next section, allows the client to have a clearer picture of how systematic reviews are structured. Beyond the

TEXTBOX 3.1. QUESTIONS TO CONSIDER DURING INITIAL REFERENCE INTERVIEW

Getting started

- What is the agreed upon definition of a systematic review?
- What role do you expect the librarian to play in the process? (expert searcher only? writing methods section? compiling bibliography? authorship?) [See chapter 11.]

Scoping the review

- Is this appropriate as a systematic review question? Would another type of review match the topic better?
- What is the scope of the review question? What are the eligibility criteria for included studies? What type of research will be included in this review (RCT, cohort, etc.)?
- What related reviews have been previously conducted on this topic?

Product of the review

- What is the purpose of the review?
- What is the expected deliverable, such as a journal article, thesis, dissertation, or guideline?
- What standard(s) will be followed for conducting or reporting the review?
- Is a protocol required to be registered? Where should it be registered?

Project and data management (covered more in chapter 4)

- Who will be on the team for the review?
- Who will be consulted?
- What is the deadline for the review?
- What software will be used for citation management, project management, coding the data, communicating, and so on?

definition of reviews, clients need to know more about the processes that will be involved as they move forward. There are various ways to educate a client about systematic reviews, including suggesting a book, a journal article about systematic review methods for their discipline or topic, suggestions for training, or providing training throughout the consultation process or workshops in the library. More options to consider are described in chapter 11.

FEASIBILITY OF THE QUESTION

The research question should be evaluated to determine if it is appropriate for a systematic review. As it drives the rest of the process, it is important to carefully and fully discuss the implications of the questions, thinking all of the steps through with a given question. In order to determine its feasibility, the purpose of the review, the research question, and eligibility criteria of included studies need to be defined, and any related reviews need to be identified and evaluated.

Purpose of the Review

Systematic reviews may be appropriate and useful at almost all stages of research on a topic, they may serve as a useful predecessor to new research, and they are themselves new primary research. Although by its nature, a systematic review is a summary of knowledge, it also contributes to new knowledge, providing a qualitative or quantitative synthesis. Systematic reviews can provide clarity and direction when there is a large amount of information, or clearly map out when there is too little information available on a topic. They can also be used to resolve discrepancies when an issue is debated or controversial. A systematic review can be a very useful tool to plan for new research or to guide the development of training materials (McKibbon 2006). Part of determining the purpose of the review is to frame the question, starting with what type of question is being asked.

Review Questions

Types of Questions

Review questions can be categorized by the overall type, as shown in table 3.2 along with examples. While it is not important to determine which category matches the question proposed by a review author, it is good to know that there is a wide range of questions that can be answered, not just the typical effectiveness type of question. For example, questions can focus

Table 3.2. Types of review questions and examples

Type of question	*Examples*
Effectiveness of an intervention (treatment/therapy/policy)	What is the effect of the nonsmoking policy in restaurants and bars on the incidence of sick days of employees due to colds, upper respiratory infections, and asthma?
Harm	Does working in a carpentry factory lead to increased incidence of asthma or upper respiratory infections?
Causation/risk factors	What are the risk factors for dropping out of college for students whose parents did not attend college?
Screening/diagnosis	Which method of diagnosis is best for Alzheimer's? What is the best method for screening for emotionally disturbed behavior in elementary school children?
Prognosis	Are dogs who have served in war zones more likely to have shortened life spans or complications?
Prevention	What are the most effective methods for preventing bullying incidents in middle school boys?
Patient/consumer/participant experience or perceptions	What are the experiences of those consumers who have a house foreclosed?
Service delivery	Does providing online database tutorials on a library website increase student satisfaction with library services?
Cost effectiveness	What are the most cost-effective ways to reduce paper waste in small to medium businesses?

on prediction—trying to predict an outcome with a set of circumstances or epidemiologic issues such as risk factors, disease distributions, comorbidities, and others. Question types can be asked by any field, such as economic evaluations or service delivery, or could apply to many fields.

Framing Questions

While clients might be more knowledgeable about the subject matter of their reference question, they are often unable to phrase questions in a manner that is useful for research. It is the librarian's responsibility to guide the client in framing the research question appropriately (White 1989). There are many ways of framing questions depending on the topic, discipline, or type of question. The most common framework for health-related topics is PICO, which stands for population, intervention, comparison, and outcome (Richardson et al., 1995). Several frameworks are listed in table 3.3, along with the areas that have utilized or published on the frameworks. The importance of the framework is that the review authors have the opportunity to clearly and specifically state the question. As everything is based on the question, it is vital to take time to carefully construct the question.

Comparing Frameworks

Looking over the frameworks, it becomes clear that there is a great deal of overlap between the various acronyms. Table 3.4 provides a comparison to put all of them in perspective starting with the Who What How (WWH) framework, which is a great place to start during the initial meeting with clients as it is open enough to fit most questions. Tables 3.4 and 3.5 are provided to increase awareness of the variety of frameworks that have been developed. Practicing with the frameworks "enables the searcher to refine strategies to suit each particular situation rather than trying to fit a search situation to a framework" (Davies 2011). The utility of the framework is to ensure that the question is scoped appropriately and provides detail on the objective, which is the start of listing the eligibility criteria.

Eligibility Criteria

The framework selected is the beginning of determining the inclusion/exclusion criteria of studies but will not speak to all characteristics required. Further criteria may need to be included depending on the framework selected such as type of study (quantitative, qualitative), setting (geography, type of organization, school), or other characteristics. When selecting study designs, it is important to consider the type of question being asked. Table 3.5 lists types of questions with ideal types of studies to be considered. To help in finalizing the criteria, an initial search is suggested.

Scoping Search for Examples Studies

Finally, initial searches will aid in further clarification of the client's research question. The search need not be perfect or comprehensive at this point. This search will serve multiple needs such as locating eligible studies that can be used as examples for eligibility criteria and estimating the number of articles expected with the final searches. Having a few studies that are known to match eligibility criteria will help in developing the search, finding index terms and keyword terms, and testing each stage of the search. If no studies are located in this initial search, this may indicate that the eligibility criteria should be adapted further (Foster 2015).

Table 3.3. Frameworks for research questions

Framework	*Stands for*	*Disciplines/type of question*
BeHEMoTh (Booth and Carroll 2015)	Be: behavior of interest H: health context (service/policy/ intervention) E: exclusions MoTh: models or theories	Questions about theories
CHIP (Shaw 2010)	Context How Issues Population	Psychology, qualitative
CIMO (Denyer and Tranfield 2009)	Context Intervention Mechanisms Outcomes	Management, business, administration
CLIP (Wildridge and Bell 2002)	Client group Location of provided service Improvement/Information/ Innovation Professionals (who provides the service?)	Librarianship, management, policy
COPES (Gibbs 2003)	Client-oriented Practical Evidence search	Social work, health care, nursing
ECLIPSE (Wildridge and Bell 2002)	Expectation Client Location Impact Professionals Service	Management, services, policy, social care
PEO (Kahn et al. 2003)	Population Exposure Outcome	Qualitative
PECODR (Dawes et al. 2007)	Patient/population/ problem Exposure Comparison Outcome Duration Results	Medicine
PESICO (Schlosser and O'Neil-Pirozzi 2007)	Person Environments Stakeholders Intervention Comparison Outcome	Augmentative and alternative communication

Framework	*Stands for*	*Disciplines/type of question*
PICO (Richardson et al. 1995)	Patient Intervention Comparison Outcome	Clinical medicine
PICO+ (Bennett and Bennett 2000)	+context, patient values, and preferences	Occupational therapy
PICOC (Petticrew & Roberts, 2006)	Context	Social sciences
PICOS (Moher et al. 2009)	Study type	Medicine
PICOT (Richardson et al. 1995)	Time	Education, health care
PICO specific to diagnostic tests (Kim et al. 2015)	Patients/participants/ population Index tests Comparator/reference tests Outcome	Diagnostic questions
PIPOH (ADAPTE Collaboration 2009)	Population Intervention Professionals Outcomes Health care setting/ context	Screening
ProPheT (Booth et al. 2016)	Problem Phenomenon of interest Time	Social sciences, qualitative, library science
SPICE (Booth 2004)	Setting Perspective Interest Comparison Evaluation	Library and information sciences
SPIDER (Cooke et al. 2012)	Sample Phenomenon of interest Design Evaluation Research type	Health, qualitative research
WWH	Who What How	

Table 3.4. Comparing potential frameworks

Framework	*Problem/population*	*Intervention/comparison*	*Results*	*Others*
WWH	Who?	What was done? (intervention, exposure, policy, phenomenon)	How does the what affect the who?	
BeHEMoTh	Behavior of interest	Health context	Models or theories	
CHIP	Population; context	Issues	How	
CLIP	Client group; location	Improvement/information/ innovation; professionals		
CIMO	Context	Intervention; mechanisms	Outcomes	
COPES (characteristics do not fit the acronym)	Client type and problem	What you might do; alternate course of action	What you want to accomplish?	
ECLIPSE	Client group; location; expectation; professionals	Service	Impact	
PEO	Population	Exposure	Outcome	
PECODR	Patient/population/problem	Exposure; Comparison; Duration	Outcome; results	
PESICO	Person; environments; stakeholders	Intervention; comparison	Outcome	
PICO	Population	Intervention; comparison	Outcome	
PICO+	Problem; context; patient values and preferences	Intervention; comparison	Outcome	
PICOC	Population; context	Intervention or exposure; Comparison	Outcome	
PICOS	Population	Intervention; comparison	Outcome	Study design
PICOT	Population	Intervention; comparison; time	Outcome	
PICO (diagnostic tests)	Patients/participants/population	Index tests comparator/reference tests	Outcome	
PIPOH	Population; professionals; health care setting/context	Intervention	Outcome	
ProPheT	Problem	Phenomenon of interest		
SPICE	Setting; perspective	Interest; comparison	Evaluation	
SPIDER	Sample; phenomenon of interest	Design	Evaluation	Research type

Table 3.5. Types of studies to consider listed by question type

Type of question	*Types of studies*
Effectiveness of an intervention/treatment/therapy	RCT > cohort > case control > case series
Harm	RCT > cohort > case control > case series
Causation	RCT > cohort > case control > case series
Screening/diagnosis	Retrospective, blind comparison to gold standard
Prognosis	Cohort > case control > case series
Prevention	RCT > cohort > case control > case series
Patient/consumer/participant experience or perceptions	Qualitative studies: most common are phenomenological, ethnographic, and grounded theory
Service delivery	RCT
Cost effectiveness	RCT > cohort > case control > case series

Source: NICE 2012. http://www.mheducation.co.uk/openup/chapters/9780335242276.pdf.

Related Reviews

Locating related reviews is an important step in determining if the question has been answered by a systematic review already, and the need to be able to place the current review in context with previous reviews. It is very useful for the client to read, annotate, and appraise the related reviews to continue developing the scope of the review (Robinson et al. 2014). Chapter 2 provides resources to locate reviews and guidance on how to appraise a systematic review. Action box 3.1 provides an exercise of how to annotate systematic reviews to determine their scope and relationship to the question under consideration.

ACTION BOX 3.1

Find several reviews on the same topic and complete the table below:

Article	Research question	Eligibility criteria	Describe search	Overall quality of methods	Answer to research question

Final Determination of Feasibility

After framing the question, determining eligibility criteria, and evaluating previous reviews, the client needs to determine if the question is viable. It is important to determine that a systematic review is appropriate for the topic before a large amount of work has been done on the project (Bates 1998). This can be done by objectively viewing the question and considering if completing the review would be feasible and ethical, if the question is appropriate and novel enough for a review, and if the results would be meaningful and effectively address the question. Several organizations have developed lists of characteristics to acknowledge when evaluating the workability of a researcher's review topic, as shown in table 3.6. The FINER list asks the author to consider if the question is feasible (do you have the resources?), interesting (who wants this question answered?), novel (is it a new question?), ethical (should you spend resources on it?), and relevant (how will this question move the field forward?) (Hulley 2007). Booth et al. developed the acronym TREAD which strongly emphasizes the need to fully consider all resources required for a review—time, resources, expertise, audience, and data. It illuminates the necessity of a well thought out review team and/or consultants who have the skills and time to devote to the project (Booth, Sutton, and Papaioannou 2016). RETREAT follows a similar pattern, asking authors to think about the review question, epistemology, time/time-frame, resources, expertise, audience, and type of data. It was specifically designed to help those planning a qualitative synthesis, and it covers the resources needed as listed in TREAD; but it also asks the authors to consider the epistemology of the approach. This means that the "reviewer should be mindful of the need

Table 3.6. Criteria for determining if question is appropriate

Acronym	*Characteristics*
FINER	Feasible
(Hulley 2007)	Interesting
	Novel
	Ethical
	Relevant
TREAD	Time
(Booth, Noyes, et al. 2016)	Resource
	Expertise
	Audience
	Data
RETREAT	Review question
	Epistemology
	Time/time-frame
	Resources
	Expertise
	Audience
	Type of data (planning a qualitative synthesis)

Source: Booth, Noyes, et al. 2016

to not violate the philosophical foundations or integrity of the qualitative primary studies" (Booth, Noyes, et al. 2016). In other words, the synthesis approach should make sense.

These acronyms highlight the many conditions which indicate that a systematic review may not be the appropriate method. If the research question does not match the systematic review method, there may be another type of review better suited for the client's question, which are detailed in chapter 1. The scope of the question needs to be appropriate for the method—too broad and the citations to sort through will be too numerous to allow time for an in-depth analysis of the selected studies, too narrow and the search will result in little or no studies. The scope should also be set to ensure that the results will be useful to all stakeholders—practitioners, researchers, policy makers, potential end users of the research, funders, and the public.

Third, if there is already a well-conducted current review, clients will need to consider changing the scope. They should find a different approach or perspective for conducting and contextualizing the review to contribute to the literature. Review authors may choose to conduct an umbrella review (systematic reviews of systematic reviews) on the reviews.

Lastly, if the client or the librarian does not have the resources to dedicate to the project, it is unlikely that it will be completed. The review author may consider conducting a rapid review, limiting some of the processes, such as searching only one or two databases, coding or appraising by a single author, or only coding a few characteristics from each study (Booth, Sutton, and Papaioannou 2016). Review authors should also consider their skill levels for completing the steps of the review and if they have the appropriate expertise or have experts that can be consulted. Additional training or consulting will increase the time required to complete the review.

OTHER TOPICS TO DISCUSS WITH THE CLIENT

Project and Data Management

An initial reference interview for a systematic review must answer more questions than an interview for a different type of reference question. A systematic review must be held to the highest research scrutiny and be documented from start to finish. Documentation on the part of the librarian should begin with the first meetings of the research team (Gore and Jones 2015). A time frame and deadline should be agreed upon as early as possible. Searches for a systematic review take far longer to generate than other reference questions, and the expectations about how much time it will take should be discussed with the systematic review team. Searches for systematic reviews will most likely result in a large number of citations, so the form of delivering the citations needs to be determined. Members of the review team may need additional training to become comfortable with the selected product. An agreement as to what databases are to be searched should also be made. The librarian is most familiar with the available databases and should make those suggestions keeping in mind that standard systematic review protocols will often have required databases specified. As systematic reviews are generally conducted by a team of researchers, for the sake of clarity, the librarian should determine to whom they should speak regarding the project (Bates 1998).

Standards

As part of the reference interview, the librarian should inquire which standard of reporting the investigators intend to use for their systematic review. There are a number of reporting guidelines published and accepted by the disciplines. These guidelines will shape the entire process of the project and should be decided upon as early as possible in the project. Many factors determine which standard the researchers should choose including the popularity of the standard, a discipline-specific standard, or a standard required for a specific journal. In the health sciences, the most popular standard is PRISMA (Preferred Reporting Items for Systematic Reviews and Meta-Analyses), but that is by no means the only accepted standard. This guideline has also been applied in other fields such as education. Chapter 10 provides details on reporting guidelines and how to apply them to the review for writing the protocol, abstract, or final product.

The Role of the Librarian

Finally, the systematic review author(s) should be in agreement as to the role of the librarian through the project. Traditionally, the librarian will handle the search and write the search methods section of the report. The librarian should request an authorship credit based on the amount and value of the work they will provide to the project (McKibbon 2006). However, if an advisory role rather than a coinvestigator one is agreed upon, either due to the needs of the patron or due to limited library time and resources, then coauthorship is not required. More details are provided in chapters 10 and 11.

CONCLUSION

The initial planning stages of the review can be difficult but with guidance can lead to starting a valuable research project. With appropriate planning, the review process can meet the needs of all involved. Further considerations, including project and data management, are discussed in the next chapter.

REFERENCES

ADAPTE Collaboration. 2009. The ADAPTE Process: Resource Toolkit Guideline Adaptation. http://www.g-i-n.net/document-store/working-groups-documents/adaptation/adapte-resource-toolkit-guideline-adaptation-2-0.pdf.

Bates, Mary Ellen. 1998. "Finding the Question behind the Question." *Information Outlook* 2 (7): 19.

Bennett, S., and J. W. Bennett. 2000. "The Process of Evidence-Based Practice in Occupational Therapy: Informing Clinical Decisions." *Australian Occupational Therapy Journal* 47 (4): 171–80.

Booth, Andrew. 2006. "Clear and Present Questions: Formulating Questions for Evidence Based Practice." *Library Hi Tech* 24 (3): 355–68.

Booth, Andrew, and Christopher Carroll. 2015. "Systematic Searching for Theory to Inform Systematic Reviews: Is It Feasible? Is It Desirable?" *Health Information and Libraries Journal* 32 (3): 220–35.

Booth, A., J. Noyes, K. Flemming, A. Gerhardus, P. Wahlster, G. J. Van Der Wilst, K. Mozygemba, et al. 2016. *Guidance on Choosing Qualitative Evidence Synthesis Methods for Use in Health Technology Assessments of Complex Interventions.* Health Technology Assessments.

Booth, Andrew, Anthea Sutton, and Diana Papaioannou. 2016. *Systematic Approaches to a Successful Literature Review*. 2nd ed. Los Angeles: Sage. https://study.sagepub.com/booth2e.

Cooke, A., D. Smith, and A. Booth. 2012. "Beyond PICO: The SPIDER Tool for Qualitative Evidence Synthesis." *Qualitative Health Research* 22 (10): 1435–43. doi:10.1177/1049732312452938.

Davies, Karen Sue. 2011. "Formulating the Evidence Based Practice Question: A Review of the Frameworks." *Evidence Based Library and Information Practice* 6 (2): 75–80. https://ejournals.library.ualberta.ca/index.php/EBLIP/article/view/9741.

Dawes, Martin, Pierre Pluye, Laura Shea, Roland Grad, Arlene Greenberg, and Jian-Yun Nie. 2007. "The Identification of Clinically Important Elements within Medical Journal Abstracts: Patient-Population-Problem, Exposure-Intervention, Comparison, Outcome, Duration and Results (PECODR)." *Informatics in Primary Care* 15 (1): 9–16.

Denyer, David, and David Tranfield. 2009. "Producing a Systematic Review." In *Sage Handbook of Organizational Research Methods*, ed. D. Buchanan and A. Bryman, 671–89. Los Angeles: Sage Publications.

Durrance, Joan C. 1995. "Factors that Influence Reference Success: What Makes Questioners Willing to Return?" *Reference Librarian* 23 (49–50): 243–65.

Foster, Margaret J. 2015. "An Overview of the Role of Librarians in Systematic Reviews: From Expert Searcher to Project Manager." *Journal of EAHIL* 11 (3): 3–7.

Gibbs, L. (2003). *Evidence Based Practice for the Helping Profession: A Practical Guide with Integrated Multimedia*. Pacific Grove, CA: Brooks/Cole-Thomson Learning.

Gore, Genevieve C., and Julie Jones. 2015. "Systematic Reviews and Librarians: A Primer for Managers." *Partnership: The Canadian Journal of Library and Information Practice and Research* 10 (1): 1–16. http://search.proquest.com/docview/1699221382.

Hulley, Stephen B. 2007. *Designing Clinical Research*. Philadelphia: Lippincott Williams and Wilkins.

Kahn, K. S., R. Kunz, J. Kleijnen, and G. Antes. 2003. *Systematic Reviews to Support Evidence-Based Medicine: How to Review and Apply Findings of Health Care Research*. London: RSM Press.

Kern, M., K. Woodward, and B. S. Woodward. 2011. "The Reference Interview." In *Reference and Information Services*, ed. Richard Bopp and Linda C. Smith, 4th ed., 57–94. Santa Barbara, CA: Libraries Unlimited.

Kim, Kyung Won, Juneyoung Lee, Sang Hyun Choi, Jimi Huh, and Seong Ho Park. 2015. "Systematic Review and Meta-Analysis of Studies Evaluating Diagnostic Test Accuracy: A Practical Review for Clinical Researchers—Part I. General Guidance and Tips." *Korean Journal of Radiology* 16 (6): 1175–87.

McKibbon, Ann. 2006. "Systematic Reviews and Librarians." *Library Trends* 55 (1): 202–15. doi:10.1353/lib.2006.0049. http://muse.jhu.edu/journals/library_trends/v055/55.1mckibbon.html.

Moher, David, Alessandro Liberati, Jennifer Tetzlaff, and Douglas G. Altman. 2009. "Preferred Reporting Items for Systematic Reviews and Meta-Analyses: The PRISMA Statement." *Annals of Internal Medicine* 151 (4): 264–69.

Petticrew, Mark, and Helen Roberts. 2006. *Systematic Reviews in the Social Sciences: A Practical Guide*. Malden, MA: Blackwell Publishers.

Richardson, W. S., M. C. Wilson, J. Nishikawa, and R. S. Hayward. 1995. "The Well-Built Clinical Question: A Key to Evidence-Based Decisions." *ACP Journal Club* 123 (3): 12.

Robinson, K. A., E. P. Whitlock, M. E. Oneil, J. K. Anderson, L. Hartling, D. M. Dryden, M. Butler, et al. 2014. "Integration of Existing Systematic Reviews into New Reviews: Identification of Guidance Needs." *Systematic Reviews* 3 (1): 60.

Schlosser, R. W., and T. O'Neil-Pirozzi. 2007. "Problem Formulation in Evidence-Based Practice and Systematic Reviews." *Contemporary Issues in Communication Sciences and Disorders* 33:5–10.

Shaw, R. L. 2010. "Conducting Literature Reviews." In *Doing Qualitative Research in Psychology: A Practical Guide*, ed. M. Forrester, 39–52. London: Sage.

Vandenberg, Laura N., Marlene Ågerstrand, Anna Beronius, Claire Beausoleil, Åke Bergman, Lisa A. Bero, Carl-Gustaf Bornehag, et al. 2016. "A Proposed Framework for the Systematic Review and Integrated Assessment (SYRINA) of Endocrine Disrupting Chemicals." *Environmental Health: A Global Access Science Source* 15 (1): 74. doi:10.1186/s12940-016-0156-6.

White, Marilyn Domas. 1989. "Different Approaches to the Reference Interview." *Reference Librarian* 11 (25–26): 631–46.

Wildridge, Valerie, and Lucy Bell. 2002. "How CLIP Became ECLIPSE: A Mnemonic to Assist in Searching for Health Policy/Management Information." *Health Information and Libraries Journal* 19 (2): 113–15.

Chapter Four

Planning the Review, Part 2

Team Dynamics and Data Management

Mark P. MacEachern, Whitney A. Townsend, and Nancy J. Allee

Project Managers are the most creative pros in the world; we have to figure out everything that could go wrong, before it does.

—Fredrik Haren

OBJECTIVES

- Define data management within a systematic review context
- Understand how data management is described in systematic review standards
- Understand the data that must be collected and managed in systematic review projects
- Understand team roles and responsibilities as they relate to systematic reviews
- Describe opportunities for librarian involvement in data management
- Learn how to use and leverage systematic review software

PROJECT AND TIME MANAGEMENT

In some cases, it is advantageous to the team if the librarian acts as the project manager, facilitating collaboration among team members and streamlining the process of the systematic review. At the very least, project management issues, such as how to manage resources, assign tasks, and divide time, must be discussed with the team. During the planning of the review, the role of the librarian must be clearly defined, and a plan for providing search results should also be detailed. The expected timeline of when deliverables will be due should be covered. Often researchers new to the systematic review process will expect a quicker turnaround than what usually happens, and when negotiating deadlines, it can be helpful to refer to Cochrane's sample timeline in section 2.3 of the *Cochrane Handbook*, which estimates twelve months at least for a review to be completed.

For the process of searching, data management issues will come into play. These will be discussed later in this chapter. During the screening process, the need for at least two independent reviewers should be communicated to the systematic review team, and a librarian can also play a role by helping pilot test the screening process for quality assurance to ensure a high interrater reliability level between reviewers. Librarians may also suggest potential software to help with the screening. Tools are also needed for the risk of bias assessment and coding. The *Cochrane Handbook* covers component lists for randomized controlled trials in section 8.5. The Joanna Briggs Institute also lists components for descriptive/case series, qualitative studies, cohort studies, and case control studies. For coding or data abstraction, there should be a unique coding form created for each review, with a list of characteristics of the studies that need to be collected, and librarians can offer examples of coding forms available from the Cochrane Collaboration and Agency for Healthcare Research Quality (AHRQ).

For the reporting process, in cases of coauthorship, it should be made clear from the beginning that the librarian will write the methods about the search strategies, as the librarian is the one most qualified to adequately describe and document the searches that were done (Foster 2015).

OVERVIEW

Data management is an important part of the systematic review process. While librarians are likely to view data management in terms of citation management, its scope within systematic reviews is far more extensive. Certainly the systematic review team needs to effectively organize and manage citations retrieved through the comprehensive database searches, but the team also needs to manage the clinical data they extract from those citations. Moreover, systematic review teams need to manage the inclusion and exclusion decisions from multiple reviewers, and manage the reviewing process in such a way that those multiple reviewers can easily review—and compare notes on—the pool of possibly relevant studies. These decisions involve hundreds and thousands of citations, *plus* reviewer screening comments about those studies, *plus* the methodological strengths and weaknesses of a good number of those studies, and so on. It's a lot of data, important data, data that are the backbone of the systematic review.

Managing the data effectively, then, is important. Standards specifically written to aid researchers with the systematic review process include recommendations on the types of data to collect but offer limited guidance on how best to manage them. Librarians are proficient organizers and licensors of information and can productively apply these skills to the relatively unsettled systematic review data management terrain. As the people most likely responsible for the comprehensive literature searches, librarians should at least be able to effectively manage the resulting citations they distribute to the team. However, that need not be the extent of the librarian's role. Librarians are uniquely positioned to suggest strategies for archiving data and licensing software designed to facilitate the review process. Small teams are unlikely to have the resources to address these concerns, which provides opportunities for librarians to stake claims in these areas. In this chapter we will define data management within the context of systematic reviews and discuss novel approaches to librarian involvement in these projects.

DEFINING DATA MANAGEMENT

Penn State University Libraries defines data management succinctly as "the process of controlling the information generated during a research project" (Penn State University Libraries 2016). Systematic reviews result in a lot of information, and it requires a process that threads through the entire project to manage it. Effective data management encompasses all aspects of the review and should include input from more than one member of the systematic review team. As a search-heavy project, the comprehensive database searches, which occur early in the project, comprise a significant portion of a systematic review's data. The person conducting the searches needs to keep track of those result numbers and all information pertaining to the searches, including databases searched, search terms and filters used, and other information needed to adequately report the searches. Inclusion and exclusion decisions also need to be managed, as does the data extraction process. If a data management plan is not in place, the systematic review is at risk for being poorly conducted and reported, which "diminishes their value to clinicians, policy makers, and other users" (Liberati et al. 2009).

GUIDELINES AND STRATEGIES FOR DATA MANAGEMENT

Data Management appears to varying degrees in the *Cochrane Handbook* and the National Academies' *Standards for Systematic Reviews* (Eden et al.

2011; Higgins and Green 2011). While specific data management resources are called out at times within the standards, there is no one resource or software tool that handles all data. For example, the *Cochrane Handbook* references their own information management system, RevMan, which serves as a template to assist Cochrane authors with their reviews, but the *Handbook* also acknowledges that other software is needed, including spreadsheets and citation management programs, such as EndNote and RefWorks. The National Academies standards also recommend the use of RevMan, EndNote, and RefWorks to assist with the documentation of the searches. The latter two programs allow investigators to collect and manage all citations from the searches, facilitating de-duplication and eligibility screening processes. Data extraction tools are necessary to handle the information gleaned from select studies identified through the searches, and these tools may be as simple as a paper form. Statistical software, like SAS, SPSS, or STATA, may also be needed for statistical components of the review.

It is unlikely that one software package will be capable of handling all data components of the review. Instead, investigators are likely to need citation management software, productivity software, statistical software, and data extraction tools. Recently, new software has entered the marketplace that is designed specifically for systematic reviews, allowing investigators to manage citations and create the tables and figures that are commonplace in systematic reviews. We discuss such software in greater detail below. Even as the market matures and the software becomes more sophisticated and able to handle data from more aspects of the review, it is important to remember that data management is a process that should occur continuously in real time.

Table 4.1. Data management recommendations

Cochrane	• Use bibliographic software and collect the following citation fields (section 6.5): ○ Abstract ○ Unique identifier ○ Author affiliations ○ Clinical trial number ○ Comments, corrections, errata, retractions, and updates ○ Index terms ○ Language of article • Use data extraction forms (section 7.5) • Use spreadsheets or database programs (section 7.8)
National Academies	• Use reference management software to handle citations and aid with documentation (section 3.4) • Manage data collection with multiple reviewers and data extraction forms (section 3.5)

WHAT INFORMATION SHOULD BE COLLECTED?

As imprecise as the standards are about data management strategies, they are as precise about the data that should be collected and reported. When conducting the searches, the investigator needs to document all aspects of the search to ensure transparent reporting. Thus, the databases searched, the dates the searches were run, any limits that were applied to the searches, and any supplemental approaches to identify possibly relevant citations—all of these need to be reported in the final manuscript. All searches should be documented and saved, perhaps in the databases themselves and in a word processor, which will help when the searches are rerun and published. Furthermore, all data needed for the PRISMA flow chart should be collected along the way. Given that the flow chart will include information from the screening process, it is important that the people involved in the searches and screening processes are aware of its inclusion at the outset of the project. See box 4.1 for a list of the information that is needed for the final manuscript.

TEXTBOX 4.1. INFORMATION FOR REPORTING SEARCHES

- Complete reproducible search strategies for publication
- Databases searched, with dates of coverage
- Dates searches were run, including the most recent if there was an update
- Limits applied (publication types, date, language)
- Grey literature sources
- Supplemental strategies (reference list checks, hand searches)
- Individuals or organizations contacted
- Number of unique citations retrieved from searches
- Number of duplicates identified
- Flowchart information
- Important decisions made while constructing searches

While librarians will primarily be conducting database searches in systematic review projects, the team will, as a whole, be responsible for collecting and managing additional data. This includes the information that derives from screening, data extraction, and statistical analyses.

WHERE TO BEGIN

As we have discussed, data management is a process that threads its way through an entire project. Data management will also involve the work of several team members. For these reasons, it is important to incorporate and discuss data management strategies as early in the project as possible, during the initial consultation or team meeting. Knowing what data to collect at the outset is integral because gathering data retrospectively is difficult and sometimes impossible. Such retrospective work can also result in poor methodology. Allocating responsibility and defining roles, then, is imperative.

TEXTBOX 4.2. BEST PRACTICES SUGGESTION

Members of the team may not realize how much search-related information there will be. Use this opportunity to educate the team about what comprehensive searching means and requires. Also listen to the needs of the team because the more you know about the project, the more helpful you can be.

TEAM COMMUNICATION AND DATA MANAGEMENT

A systematic review team may be as small as two people, or involve dozens of individuals across the globe. Most, if not all, of these individuals will be interacting with the systematic review data in some way. Because of this complexity, systematic reviews require a team approach in order to adhere to appropriate methodology and existing professional standards. In our experience, successful teams have effective communication at all stages of the review, including those that involve data management.

Ideally, open communication will begin to develop as early as the protocol. At that point, a large dispersed team may divide into task-based subgroups and rarely communicate as a full membership, while smaller teams may use regular face-to-face interactions to share information and stay on track. Whatever the team makeup, it is important to establish strong communication with at least the person(s) you will be working with most closely. It is also important to communicate with others on the team so that you know, as the person who will be providing the search results to those doing the screening, how the screening will be done and what the team's software preferences are.

You want to be sure to provide the citations in a format that will facilitate the screening and other processes.

Communicating realistic timelines is also important, because unrealistic timelines doom many systematic review projects. Team members may not fully grasp that reviews can take upwards of a year or more to complete. They also might not appreciate the length of time it takes to conduct comprehensive searches in multiple databases and manage the unusually large result sets. Furthermore, librarians may easily underestimate the amount of time it takes to export citations from databases to the bibliographic software, perform the de-duplication processes, and put the citations in a workable format for the other team members. Indeed, data management can add significant time to the search process, which the entire team should discuss and expect as they embark on the project.

TEAM ROLES AND DATA MANAGEMENT

While some individuals may come in for a search consultation with plans of conducting a systematic review alone, they should be encouraged to expand their team to include others with differing skill sets to better adhere to the standards. Ideally, a suitable team is established early in the process, consisting of at least two members so as to minimize the possibility that bias negatively impacts the review. Given that there are many components to a systematic review, some team members may take on more than one role. These roles include the following (see table 4.2):

- Content or clinical expert
- Methods and research design expert
- Librarian or search expert
- Statistician
- Data manager
- Consumers and stakeholders

Content or Clinical Expert

Content experts are generally defined as clinicians or researchers with significant knowledge of the question under review. Content experts help define the topic and are generally involved throughout the entire research process, particularly with eligibility screening. Ideally, there are at least two content experts on the team so that certain aspects of the review can be completed by more than one person.

Table 4.2. Team composition recommendations

Organization	*Recommendations*
Cochrane (section 2.3.4)	• Topic expert • Methods expert • Statistician • Consumers
National Academies (section 2.1)	• Clinical expert • Methods expert • Librarian or search expert • Other expertise as appropriate
Joanna Briggs	• Methods expert • Content expert • Consumers and stakeholders • Search expert
Campbell Collaboration	• Methods and research design expert • Search expert • Content expert • Statistician • Data management knowledge

Methods and Research Design Experts

At least one member of the team should have expertise with systematic review methodology to ensure that the appropriate methods are followed throughout the review. A thorough knowledge of primary research methodology is critical to designing the screening, appraisal, and data extraction steps. While not all librarians will work in this capacity, they can contribute to improved methods by pointing teams to the appropriate standards and ensuring that their own searches meet those standards. In fact, there is evidence to show that inclusion of a librarian on a systematic review team increases adherence to search-related reporting standards (Koffel 2015; Rethlefsen et al. 2015).

Librarian or Search Expert

The studies identified through the search process are the foundation of every systematic review, and a librarian or someone equally qualified to conduct the comprehensive searches should be involved in the project. The person(s) responsible for the searches should (1) consider software for the management of all the information and data collected throughout the search process, and (2) be familiar with the file formats and programs needed by those doing the eligibility screening. Depending on the program, the searcher may choose to hide certain pieces of citation information from the screeners, such as authors and journal titles, so as to minimize the likelihood that that information influences screening decisions.

Statistician

The involvement of a statistician is often recommended to advise on and perform statistical measures, tests for heterogeneity, and tests for bias and to present the results using appropriate graphs and data visualization tools. Statisticians may need to use specialized software to handle the calculations.

Data Management Expert

At least one member of the team, usually the project lead, should be prepared to manage the flow of data throughout the entire review process. Much of the initial data are citations, but that quickly extends into all the succeeding steps along the way, from selecting studies to analyzing results. This requires the data manager to be familiar with a variety of files, programs, and software and to manage them in such a way that data can be effectively retrieved at any point during and after the review.

Consumers and Stakeholders

Many organizations also see value in including stakeholders on a systematic review team to help prioritize questions and provide different perspectives on issues related to the review topic. Such individuals or groups can include consumers (patients), institutional or government agencies, researchers, and others in health care whose perspective may provide insight into almost any aspect of the review (Cottrell et al. 2014).

DEFINING YOUR ROLE

Depending on the makeup of the team and the individual skills of each team member, librarians may be encouraged to take on new roles and responsibilities. At a minimum, librarians construct comprehensive database searches and provide researchers with the citations that are the foundation of the review. Citation management is a natural extension of the searches, so the use of bibliographic software may be the extent to which most librarians are involved in data management. However, librarians are uniquely positioned to educate team members about standards, recommend programs and appropriate software, and contribute to the larger data management needs of the

Table 4.3. Team member knowledge and responsibilities

Step	*Knowledge and skills*	*Team members*
Plan: Formulating the question and protocol	Subject-specific content Question formulation	Content expert Stakeholders Methods expert Search expert
Identifying the literature	Advanced knowledge of literature databases Advanced search skills Knowledge of grey literature resources Reference management	Content expert Search expert Data manager
Evaluate: Screening and appraisal	Subject-specific expertise Understanding of eligibility criteria Knowledge of study design and appraisal Reference/data management	Content expert Data manager Methods expert
Coding and explaining: Data extraction and analysis	Data management Knowledge of data extraction tools Appropriate statistical analysis Bias assessment	Statistician Data manager Methods expert
Summarize: Reporting and disseminating	Knowledge of reporting standards Ability to describe contributions to the review Understanding of the methods and results of the review	All

team. As new systematic review software tools become available and more commonplace in research environments, libraries and librarians may be able to leverage their neutral positions and stake a claim in the burgeoning area of systematic review technology.

SOFTWARE TOOLS FOR MANAGING SYSTEMATIC REVIEWS

Systematic reviews benefit from the use of software tools to manage the process. These tools can help streamline the steps involved in carrying out the review and assist team members in carrying out the review functions. There are several advantages to the use of systematic review software. It can make the review process more efficient by helping with data management from start to finish, from uploading articles for title-abstract screening, to appraisal of inclusion and exclusion criteria, to conducting full-text article reviews, extracting data, and analyzing results. Most software is designed to conveniently manage the importing and de-duplication of citations from search

Table 4.4. Advantages of systematic review software

Efficiency	Provides specialized functions which maximize efficiency in conducting and managing systematic reviews
Process management	Helps manage the review process from A to Z, from title and abstract review to data extraction and analysis to results and findings
Report generation	Generates reports for monitoring and tracking progress
Quality	Helps ensure consistency in adherence to systematic reviews standards
Librarian partnerships	Can facilitate ongoing librarian involvement and collaborative partnerships with systematic review teams, if software is provided as part of library services and resources

results conducted in multiple databases as well as title-abstract and full-text article screening by multiple reviewers on the review team. It also enables the creation of forms for the appraisal of inclusion and exclusion criteria for different levels of the review. Additionally, the software can generate a number of reports for monitoring the process, including PRISMA reports, article review tracking status, as well as other useful reports for data management.

The specialized software for systematic reviews allows for easy assignment of title-abstract citations and full-text articles to individual reviewers by reference identification numbers assigned to each article within the system. Team members' contributions to the review process are evident from the reports, identifying progress by individual reviewer, and these status reports are useful to overall project management and balancing the review workload of team members. The software tools help in maintaining quality assurance in the review process by identifying any areas of conflict in review decisions and by ensuring consistency in adhering to standards. Some libraries make available specialized systematic review software as part of library services and resources, providing partnership opportunities for librarians to participate on systematic reviews. As experts in the process of conducting systematic reviews, combined with expertise in using systematic review software, librarians can play a valuable role on systematic review teams.

EVALUATING SYSTEMATIC REVIEW SOFTWARE

Decisions about what specific software to use to facilitate systematic reviews should be made early on in the process. Careful thought needs to be given to the key features and functionality that are required by the review team. Table 4.5 identifies some of the criteria important to evaluate for data management of the systematic review. The list of software is not comprehensive, but it

Table 4.5. Chart of selected systematic review software key features

Software program	*Citation importing from multiple platforms*	*Screening*	*Multiple reviewers at same time*	*Multiple levels of review*	*Data reporting, analysis, and extraction*	*Data backup and security*	*Free vs. fee-based*
Abstrackr, http://abstrackr.cebm.brown.edu	✔	title-abstract	✔				free
Covidence, https://www.covidence.org	✔	title-abstract full-text/pdf	✔	✔	✔		varies: some features are provided free; some are fee-based subscription services
DistillerSR, https://distillercer.com	✔	title-abstract full-text/pdf	✔	✔	✔	✔	fee-based
EPPI-Reviewer 4, http://eppi.ioe.ac.uk/cms/er4	✔	title-abstract full-text/pdf	✔	✔	✔	✔	fee-based
Rayyan, https://rayyan.qcri.org	✔	title-abstract full-text/pdf	✔	✔			free
SUMARI, http://www.joannabriggs.org/sumari.html	✔	full-text	✔	✔	✔		fee-based

covers resources that tend to focus on managing the full range of the review process rather than focusing on only one or more narrowly defined aspects. As evident from the chart, even though free software is available, more features and functionality are offered on a fee-based, paid subscription option.

Most software is web based and allows for importing of citation data from multiple platforms, such as EndNote, PubMed, and RefWorks as well as screening of full-text articles by multiple members of the review team simultaneously. Additionally, most of the software resources allow multiple levels of review in appraising inclusion and exclusion protocols. Report generation is another important feature for data management in order to produce summary reports, such as PRISMA flow diagrams and documenting decision making. While many commonalities exist between the software sources, unique features and functionality can be helpful in determining which source is the best fit for review teams. For example, if both quantitative and qualitative data analysis are of interest, one of the characteristics of EPPI Reviewer 4 is the capability of calculating common measures of effect, such as odds ratios, risk ratios, and risk differences, as well as statistical measures, such as standard deviations and confidence intervals, in addition to allowing thematic, conceptual analysis of data.

Data backup and security are not guaranteed by all software sources. DistillerSR and EPPI Reviewer 4 provide data backup and security. Covidence, however, gives users warning that their platform is provided on an "as is" and "as available" basis, stating on their website, "We do not guarantee that use of it will be uninterrupted, timely, secure or error-free" (Covidence 2016).

ACTION BOX 4.1. IDEAL FEATURES OF DATA MANAGEMENT SOFTWARE

List the ideal features of a piece of systematic review data management software specific to your team's needs. What existing tool do you think will best fit the bill?

SOFTWARE LICENSING

In deciding whether to license fee-based specialized systematic review software, there are a number of factors to weigh. Available funding and associated costs are important considerations. It is also necessary to inquire about the review team members' interest in and willingness to learn to use new and specialized software resources versus making it work with more familiar and readily available tools and resources for data management. The time needed to acquire and implement the software, set up user accounts, and provide training for the review team lengthens the systematic review, so the overall timeline should be adjusted to account for these additional steps.

The checklist in table 4.6 provides a question set pertaining to cost, account management, training, and technical support to inquire about when licensing systematic review software. One of the most critical issues when deciding which technologies and software resources to purchase is what kind of backup is provided for data. Not all of the currently available systematic review software packages provide robust security and backup of data. Knowledge of these licensing considerations; familiarity with the functionality and key features of specialized systematic review software, in particular, data management capabilities; as well as awareness of the time and effort involved in integrating new software resources into the systematic review process are examples of other valuable roles librarians can provide in consulting and advising about the management of systematic reviews.

Table 4.6. Licensing and user agreement checklist

Cost	
Is an educational discount offered?	Yes/No
Are there different rates by user category, e.g., faculty, student, other?	Yes/No
As number of user accounts increases, does cost per user account decrease, e.g., $120/month for 50–10 users, $100/month for 11–20 users?	Yes/No
Are monthly accounts offered?	Yes/No
Account management	
Are unlimited project sites available per user account?	Yes/No
Is information provided on confidentiality and privacy regarding user accounts and data?	Yes/No
Is multi-institutional project work by review teams supported?	Yes/No
Training	
Is training provided for project administrators and user support team?	Yes/No
Is training provided for systematic review team members?	Yes/No
Are there limits on number of training sessions during the contract period?	Yes/No
Is training available on one-time, train-the-trainer, or ongoing basis?	Yes/No
Technical support	
Is technical support available 24×7?	Yes/No
Is technical support provided free of charge?	Yes/No
Backup and maintenance	
Is information on policies and procedures for security and backup of data provided?	Yes/No
Is information on maintenance protocols and routines provided?	Yes/No

TECHNICAL AND USER SUPPORT

In addition to team roles discussed earlier that are necessary for handling the systematic review, technical and user support are also important functions. Technical support is typically provided as part of the licensing for fee-based software, but it may not be as directly accessible for other available software. The review team may want to designate a point person, as project administrator, to have lead on interfacing with technical support for addressing questions and issues that arise in the review process.

User support is needed too as an interface between review team members and system technical support for a variety of functions, including managing user accounts, setting up new project sites, importing citations, creating appraisal forms, generating reports, and other data management processes. Training review team members on the software may also need to be provided if the review team is using it for the first time. Training may include holding webinars or video-conferencing sessions for user support as well as developing online tutorials and videos for ongoing training needs if these resources are not provided. Review team membership may change during the systematic review process, so training may need to be offered at various points throughout completion of the project.

CONCLUSION

There is growing demand for systematic reviews. In health-related disciplines, they set a gold standard for comprehensively and systematically reviewing the research literature on topics of interest, adhering to well-defined standards, and synthesizing the results into a well-informed, evidence-based assessment. They form the basis of health-care guidelines and contribute to health policy. As the emphasis on health-care quality, patient safety, and cost effectiveness drives decision making, the demand for systematic reviews will continue to increase.

The technique for conducting systematic reviews is applicable beyond health sciences disciplines, however, and there is also growing interest in using this method for conducting in-depth reviews of the literature in other disciplines. While faculty, researchers, and clinicians have content knowledge, they may lack experience in conducting the steps involved in systematic reviews and managing the full review process. Librarians have this expertise and have increasingly expanded roles beyond providing consultations, developing search strategies, and executing searches in relevant databases. Librarians have the necessary skills to actively participate on systematic review teams in a number of valuable roles: advising on methodology, determining criteria for inclusion and exclusion, extracting data, and analyzing results as well as selecting software for data management. There are new opportunities for collaboration on systematic review teams, including interinstitutional collaboratives and global partnerships that provide best evidence reviews of the research literature and for a variety of professional development initiatives, including creation of continuing education courses and other training resources for librarians as well as discipline-focused faculty development workshops. Librarians can also play a role in software development for systematic reviews by conducting comparative evaluations of system features and functionality and advising review teams about which software will best meet the team's information and data management needs.

REFERENCES

Campbell Collaboration. "Producing a Review." Accessed February 2, 2016. http://www.campbellcollaboration.org/systematic_reviews/index.php.

Cottrell, E., E. Whitlock, E. Kato, S. Uhl, S. Belinson, C. Chang, T. Hoomans, D. Meltzer, H. Noorani, K. Robinson, M. Schoelles, M. Motu-apuaka, J. Anderson, R. Paynter, and J. M. Guise. 2014. "Defining the Benefits of Stakeholder Engagement in Systematic Reviews." *AHRQ Methods for Effective Health Care*. http://www.ncbi.nlm.nih.gov/pubmedhealth/PMH0077182.

Covidence. "Platform Availability and Changes." Accessed February 2, 2016. https://www.covidence.org/terms.

Eden, J., L. Levit, A. Berg, and S. Morton, eds. 2011. *Finding What Works in Health Care: Standards for Systematic Reviews*. Washington, DC: National Academies Press.

Foster, M. J. 2015. "An overview of the role of librarians in systematic reviews: from expert search to project manager." *Journal of EAHIL* 11(3):3–7.

Higgins, J. P. T., and S. Green, eds. 2011. *Cochrane Handbook for Systematic Reviews of Interventions*. Version 5.1.0. The Cochrane Collaboration. Available from www.cochrane-handbook.org.

Joanna Briggs Institute. 2015. *The Joanna Briggs Institute Method for Systematic Review Research Quick Reference Guide.* Accessed February 2, 2016. http://www.joannabriggs.org/assets/docs/jbc/operations/can-synthesise/CAN_SYNTH SISE_Resource-V4.pdf.

Koffel, J. B. 2015. "Use of Recommended Search Strategies in Systematic Reviews and the Impact of Librarian Involvement: A Cross-Sectional Survey of Recent Authors." *PLoS One* 10 (5): e0125931.

Liberati, A., D. G. Altman, J. Tetzlaff, C. Mulrow, P. C. Gøtzsche, et al. 2009. "The PRISMA Statement for Reporting Systematic Reviews and Meta-Analyses of Studies That Evaluate Health Care Interventions: Explanation and Elaboration." *PLoS Medicine* 6 (7): e1000100. doi:10.1371/journal.pmed.1000100.

Penn State University Libraries. "What Is Data Management?" Accessed February 2, 2016. https://www.libraries.psu.edu/psul/pubcur/what_is_dm.html.

Rethlefsen, M. L., A. M. Farrell, T. L. C. Osterhaus, and T. J. Brigham. 2015. "Librarian Co-authors Correlated with Higher Quality Reported Search Strategies in General Internal Medicine Systematic Reviews." *Journal of Clinical Epidemiology* 68 (6): 617–26.

Chapter Five

Identifying the Studies, Part 1

Database Searching

Susan Fowler

Google can bring you back 100,000 answers. A librarian can bring you back the right one.

—Neil Gaiman

OBJECTIVES

- Understand methods for choosing databases
- Understand methods and issues in designing search strategies

OVERVIEW

Systematic reviews require systematic searching. The process of choosing databases should be thorough and their choices intentional. To be systematic the decisions we make about how we design search strategies should be based on evidence. There are, at minimum, four types of searches in a systematic review: preliminary; exhaustive database; hand search; and contacting experts.

A preliminary search is the first search conducted in the review. The goal of a preliminary search is to identify existing reviews on the topic of interest, assess the volume of potentially relevant studies, and locate a minimum of two to four articles to use as example articles. Those example articles can help the librarian design an exhaustive database search. The goal of an exhaustive database search is to identify as many publications as possible that meet the requirement of the review. This chapter will discuss the best methods for choosing databases and designing exhaustive database search strategies based on available evidence.

Table 5.1. Four types of searches in a systematic review

Type of search	*Purpose*	*Sources*	*Document*	*Skill level*
Preliminary	Identify existing reviews Assess volume of potentially relevant studies Locate at least 2–4 example articles that meet your review criteria	Scopus Cochrane Library PubMed	Sources searched and terms used for research notes and to share with librarian	Medium
Exhaustive database	Identify all publications and as much grey literature as possible that meet study requirements	Scopus Cochrane Library Ovid Medline Embase CINAHL Subject-specific databases Trial registries	*Sources and platforms *Dates *Applied database supplied limits * # of search results * Completely replicable search * = required for reporting in publications	Advanced
Hand search	Identify grey literature like conference proceedings, abstracts for posters, and presented papers not indexed in online databases	Subject-specific professional association websites Major relevant journals Bibliographies of all included studies Bibliographies of on-topic reviews	*Sources searched *Dates *# of search results * = required for reporting in publications	Medium
Contact experts	Identify unregistered studies with unpublished results or potential results		Names, dates, and methods of contact All responses	

CHOOSING DATABASES

There are so many databases available it can be daunting to consider the task of choosing the right ones for a particular systematic review. At the same time, if the librarian has some favorite databases, it is easy to make the mistake of defaulting to those without considering that others may offer citations not indexed in their defaults.

Choice of database can impact the performance of a search. In information retrieval research, two measurements used to determine search performance are precision and recall. Precision is the number of items that are relevant out of the total number of items a search retrieved. Precision is measured against the search results. Recall is the total number of relevant items a search retrieved out of the total number of relevant items in the database. Recall is, in theory, measured against the database. In reality, knowing the context of all content in a database is not realistic. In practice, precision and recall are measured against a pool of studies from within a database. For example, to develop an optimal search strategy for detecting clinically relevant qualitative studies in Medline, Wong and team first developed a pool to test the search against. They developed the pool by reviewing and classifying all articles within a set of journals and years. Having this pool allowed them to then run the search they had designed against the pool to determine the precision and recall performance of the search (Wong, Wilczynski, and Haynes 2004). It isn't necessary or feasible to measure precision and recall for every search a librarian designs for a systematic review, but understanding these concepts and how they contribute to the overall science of information retrieval is useful when choosing databases and designing exhaustive searches. In an exhaustive database search, the goal is to not miss any relevant items that exist in the database, therefore achieving high recall. In choosing databases, consider how the database will impact recall and precision. Searching more than one database for a systematic review is essential. In an oft-cited study by Gavel and Iselid of four databases, all four had some overlap while all four also had unique content (Gavel and Iselid 2008). Guidelines like the *Preferred Reporting Items for Systematic Reviews and Meta-Analyses* (PRISMA) and the National Academies' *Standards for Systematic Reviews* recommend searching more than one database as part of increasing recall and decreasing the potential for bias (Moher et al. 2015; Morton et al. 2011). The librarian is the database expert of a research team. It is up to them to know databases well enough to choose databases intentionally and to explain those choices. The librarian may be working with a researcher who wants to use a "database" that is not really a database, or the researcher may want the librarian to use a resource they do not fully understand themselves and it will be up to the librarian to explain the resulting content. For example, a member of the research team may want to use Google Scholar. While Google Scholar has many benefits, including the ability to search through full text, it is not a good resource for systematic reviews. Google Scholar will not disclose the algorithm by which search results are ordered, making it impossible to create search strategies in Google Scholar that are replicable (Haddaway et al. 2015). As the search expert, it falls on the librarian to explain this to the rest of the research team. When choosing databases, the librarian should do some research first. Some questions to ask when considering each database include the following:

- Are the topics in the research question covered?
- What types of materials are indexed?
- Is this the only and/or best platform to this database?

All of this information is usually in the About section of the database website.

To begin the process of choosing databases by subject, it is good to start with the example articles located in the preliminary search. Find out the databases in which those example articles have been indexed. Another good way to find subject databases is on library websites that include discovery tools which list databases by subject. If the review is on a topic outside your normal area of focus, you may consider contacting a special library or librarian in that field for recommendations. And finally, your researchers may have suggestions about databases specific to their field.

Databases index more than published research articles. Databases index all sorts of materials, for example, current or completed but unpublished clinical trials, chemical abstracts, dissertations, and even DNA. Three examples of databases that include materials outside of published research articles are ProQuest Dissertations & Theses (PQDT), the Cochrane Central Register of Controlled Trials (CENTRAL), and ClinicalTrials.gov. PQDT indexes dissertations. Dissertations often include primary research and original ideas that are not accessible anywhere else. Dissertations have the added benefit of large bibliographies that can be searched for additional resources (ProQuest 2016). CENTRAL is a database of reports of randomized clinical trials and controlled clinical trials. It includes records pulled from Medline and Embase automatically, but it also includes poster and paper abstracts identified through hand searching conference proceedings which may never become published journal articles and content in published journals that won't be indexed in any other database (Higgins and Green 2011). Locating and using such materials can decrease bias in the review, but it is also possible that abstracts will not have enough information to meet the inclusion criteria for analysis. ClinicalTrials.gov is a trials registry that includes both government and privately funded trials. Several of the trials are ongoing. While the data for an ongoing trial may not yet be available, it is useful for your team members to know that a trial in their topic area is ongoing and that the results, once concluded, may change the results of the systematic review. This information can be communicated in the discussion section of the manuscript. When the trials are completed, the files in ClinicalTrials.gov are updated to include the results. This allows us to see results whether or not the study will ever be published as an article. Again, including this material in a review decreases bias.

A platform is the user interface to a database. Platforms can vary in the search tools available, which in turn can affect the precision and recall performance of a search strategy. The types and timeliness of materials retrieved is also affected by the platform. A well-known and widely used database in medicine is the Medical Literature Analysis and Retrieval System Online also known as Medline. Medline indexes citations and abstracts from academic journals on topics in medicine, allied health, and biological sciences (U.S. National Library of Medicine 2015b). Medline is freely available and searchable online and through many platforms, including but not limited to PubMed, Ovid, EBSCO, Embase, Scopus, and TRIP. Some platforms, like PubMed and TRIP, search and produce records from more sources than just Medline, which can increase the recall and decrease bias of a search. Other platforms like Ovid and EBSCO provide advanced search tools not available in PubMed or TRIP that can increase the precision of a search.

It is important the librarian understand what databases and platforms they choose and to have well informed reasons for those choices. The librarian does not have to limit their choice to just one platform of each database. Since the differences in platforms can impact search results, it can be good to search more than one. It is also important to track what tools, platforms, and databases are searched, since that information is often required by reporting guidelines such as PRISMA (Moher et al. 2015). More information about PRISMA is available in chapter 9. In addition to searching more than one platform, standard guidelines require searching more than one database, and choice of databases should be thoughtful and well informed.

DESIGNING THE SEARCH STRATEGY

A systematic review on the effectiveness of medical interventions "attempts to collate all empirical evidence that fits pre-specified eligibility criteria in order to answer a specific research question" (Higgins and Green 2011). Collating all the evidence for a systematic review requires designing thorough and expert search strategies in a systematic way that err on the side of recall. Thoroughness involves term harvesting, considering previously constructed and validated search filters, and searching across several databases. Expert searchers have a fundamental understanding of what is indexed in the databases they are searching and know the best tools to use to search those databases. A systematic approach involves designing search strategies across databases as similarly as possible, keeping notes about why decisions were made along the way and tracking all the search strategies in such a way that they can be reproduced with the same results by an independent party months or years later.

The Canadian Agency of Drugs and Technologies in Health conducted an in-depth study that included a systematic review, web-based survey, and peer-review forums to determine the most important methods for designing exhaustive database searches. Their work revealed various search tools and methods as well as common mistakes that can have a significant impact on search results. A result of their work is an evidence-based tool to review search strategies called PRESS (Peer Review of Electronic Search Strategies) (Sampson et al. 2008). The PRESS tool serves as an excellent framework when considering all the elements of designing a search strategy. PRESS highlights errors most commonly found in systematic review search strategies for peer reviewers to check including conceptualization of the research question, spelling errors, translation of search strategy across databases, appropriate inclusion of subject headings, and appropriate inclusion of natural language, spelling variants and truncation, and applied search limits.

Translation of the Research Question into a Search Plan

A search plan identifies the concepts of the research question and how those concepts will be combined. Question frameworks help searchers and researchers consider and determine the important concepts of their research question. PICO is a framework for clinical medicine questions. Booth et al. found that using the PICO framework to form questions and plan a search strategy increased the precision of those searches (Booth, O'Rourke, and Ford 2000). In PICO, each letter represents an essential concept in the search, where P = patient, problem, or population; I = intervention of interest; C = comparison, which is not always applicable; and O = outcome. Box 5.1 gives an example of applying the PICO framework.

TEXTBOX 5.1. TRANSLATING A RESEARCH QUESTION INTO THE PICO FRAMEWORK

Q: Researcher wants to compare the effectiveness of weight loss versus continuous positive airway pressure on blood pressure in patients with sleep apnea.

Translated into PICO:

P = sleep apnea

I = continuous positive airway pressure

C = weight loss

O = hypertension

The most common errors in translating a research question into a search plan include missing an important concept and adding too many concepts. Missing a concept can make a search too broad. For example, from the above PICO question, if the search plan is "sleep apnea AND (continuous positive airway pressure OR weight loss)," then such a search will retrieve articles that touch on hypertension, but it will also include articles that say nothing about hypertension. Such a plan is needlessly broad. A search that adds too many concepts can either be too broad or too narrow depending on which Boolean operators are used to combine the concepts. Either way, adding concepts to the search plan that are not part of the research question will negatively impact search performance.

Boolean

Boolean is a logic tool that allows searchers to combine terms and concepts in searches to expand and reduce search results. The operator *OR* will expand the search and should be used to connect synonyms and controlled vocabulary representing the same concept, thus expanding the search for that concept. The operator *AND* should be used to combine each concept, thus limiting search results to items where all concepts are present. See box 5.2 for how this applies to our previous example.

Errors in applying Boolean operators and, more often, forgetting to use them are common. Most databases will assume an *AND* when an operator is missing, which will greatly reduce the recall and precision of your search. Searchers should apply a critical eye to their search strategy and check the Boolean operators. Finally, Boolean operators should always be capitalized. It does not matter in all database platforms, but when it does, it matters a lot. For example, in PubMed, lowercase Boolean operators are ignored and an *AND* between each term is automatically applied (Port 1997).

TEXTBOX 5.2. TRANSLATING PICO INTO A SEARCH STRATEGY

P AND (I OR C) AND O
(sleep apnea OR sleep apnoea OR sleep disordered breathing)
AND
(weight loss OR continuous positive airway pressure)
AND
(hypertension OR high blood pressure)

Term Harvesting

For systematic review research, a best practice for designing search strategies includes applying both natural language terms and controlled vocabulary, also referred to as index terms, to err on the side of recall (Sampson et al. 2009). Term harvesting refers to the process of locating all terminology expressing each concept in the research question. Term harvesting is the part of systematic review work that librarians tend to enjoy the most. The hunt can be thrilling, interesting, and offer opportunities to learn. No one can think of every term that represents a concept off the top of their heads. For that reason, it is important to take steps to be sure all possible terms have been located. There are two approaches to harvesting terms formally described in available literature: objective and conceptual. The objective approach involves mining controlled vocabulary and natural language terms from articles already known to fit the context of the research question. These are the example articles located in the preliminary search. Next, the search must be constructed objectively to see if it retrieves the known articles (Hausner et al. 2015). The conceptual approach involves using database thesauri and other resources to locate terminology related to concepts in the research question (Hausner et al. 2012). This chapter recommends using a combination of both approaches.

To harvest terms for each concept in the search, the example articles located in the preliminary search are usually the best place to start. For an efficient approach, look at each of the example articles as they are cited in each database with the title, abstract, and controlled vocabulary. Note controlled vocabulary and natural language used to address each concept in the research question and whether each example article covers all concepts in the research question. If an example article does not cover one of the essential elements of the search question, this should be investigated and resolved. It is possible that the researcher will change their question or that the librarian will need to change the essential concepts of the search.

Whether or not every term located should be used is something for which there are varying opinions among experts. What if a term representing a concept in the research question returns zero results? Should search designers leave it out of the search? Realistically the term could be left out with no ill effect; however, another school of thought is that the term may bring up results in the future when a search is redone to update the review. As long as a term doesn't bring up irrelevant results, it doesn't really matter outside of the visual aesthetic of the search.

Controlled Vocabulary

Controlled vocabulary is a list of terms under which items in a database are indexed. For example, if you are searching the PubMed platform to Medline and want all articles that have been indexed under breast cancer, you would enter *"Breast Neoplasms"[Mesh]* in the search box. Use of controlled vocabularies in searching has been widely shown to improve recall of search results (Sampson et al. 2008). Examples of controlled vocabulary include MeSH in Medline, Emtree in Embase, Subject Headings in CINAHL and ERIC, and Subject Terms in PsycINFO.

To locate controlled vocabulary terms for the concepts in the research question, start with the database citation records for each example article located during the preliminary search. Look at the controlled vocabulary the citation has been indexed under and note terms that represent each concept of the search. Controlled vocabulary will not always be the same from one database to the next. For this reason, it is best to look at how the example article was indexed in each database the team intends to search so that the librarian can apply the correct controlled vocabulary for that database. Significant differences in controlled vocabulary should be recorded in the research notes. After the librarian has gathered all related controlled vocabulary from the example articles, they should be sure to run an independent search in the thesauri of each database to be sure they have captured all possible controlled vocabulary terms.

Not all databases index items with controlled vocabulary. Scopus is an example of a database that does not index items using controlled vocabulary. Scopus, does, however, list the controlled vocabulary that items were indexed under in the Medline and Embase databases. Some databases do not use their own controlled vocabulary but do use the controlled vocabulary of other databases. For example, some records in the Cochrane Database of Systematic Reviews, Cochrane Central Register of Controlled Trials, Database of Abstracts of Reviews of Effects, Health Technology Assessments, and Economic Evaluations are indexed with Medline's MeSH controlled vocabulary (Wiley 2012).

Subheadings

Subheadings are traditionally used to further refine a search concept. For example, if the goal is to find papers in PubMed on surgery in breast cancer, it makes sense to apply the subheading of surgery to the controlled vocabulary term for breast cancer, *"Breast Neoplasms/surgery"[Mesh]*. However, Wright et al. found that use of subheadings reduces recall of a search by over 30 percent (Wright et al. 1991). Since the goal of an exhaustive search is to have a high level of recall, it is better to use floating subheadings instead, such as *"Breast Neoplasms"[Mesh] AND "surgery" [Subheading]*. Lists of floating subheadings and instructions on how to apply proper syntax are available in the Help section of most database platform websites. For example, in PubMed, floating subheadings are denoted with the word "subheading" within brackets following the actual subheading. That same subheading appears as *su.fs.* in Ovid Medline, *'surgery'/lnk* in Embase, and *[mh /SU]* in Cochrane.

Natural Language

Natural language, also commonly referred to as *text words* or *free words*, refers to noncontrolled vocabulary, the natural language, used by authors to write their manuscripts. "In a review of searches for RCTs, Dickersin, Scherer, and Lefebvre found that the limited use of text word searching was the most consistent defect" (Sampson et al. 2008). As useful as using controlled vocabulary can be, using controlled vocabulary alone can reduce recall, causing searchers to miss a significant number of publications. There are a few reasons for this. Whether records are indexed by humans or a machine, indexing isn't perfect, mistakes are made, and important concepts are missed. Sometimes there is not enough information supplied by the author to determine how an article should be indexed. There is also the issue of time. Medline records are indexed by humans, which can take anywhere from two to three months or more to complete (Silverman et al. 2005). Cochrane systematic reviews are not indexed in Cochrane for up to six months after publication (Wiley 2012). Some records in Medline never have MeSH terms applied, including conference abstracts. While new MeSH terms are continually added, older journal articles are not updated with the new MeSH terms (U.S. National Library of Medicine 2015a). Searching using natural language terms can ameliorate issues with controlled vocabulary and increase the search strategy recall.

Natural language terms can be located from many sources. The best place to start is with the example articles located through the preliminary search. Look through the title and abstract for each example article and note natural language terms and phrases used to express each concept in the research question. Other places to look for natural language terms include the records for controlled vocabulary terms which often include a list of synonyms, dictionaries, thesauri, books, and encyclopedias.

Most database platforms search natural language terms in the title and abstract fields of the citation record. Some databases will also search natural language found in the affiliation and author keywords fields of the citation records. For example, if the search the librarian is designing is about cancer, an article that has been written by authors affiliated with the National Cancer Institute but that is not about cancer will be retrieved by the search anyway. Finally, some database platforms will attempt to automatically match natural language terms to controlled vocabulary and will return search results based on that attempt. Automatic term mapping can lead to errors in context. For example, *nursing* in PubMed will be automatically matched with MeSH terms for *nursing* and also for *breast feeding*. Because of various fields in the citation record and automatic term mapping, it is best to specify the fields in which you want those terms to be searched when using natural language terms.

Truncation and Wildcards

Truncation allows searchers to search root words with various endings. For example, instead of searching just the word *compute*, adding a truncation symbol like *compute** will also return results with *computer*, *computers*, and *computerization*.

Wildcards are similar to truncation, but they work at the beginning or in the middle of terms to search variants. For example, *wom*n* will return *woman* and *women*.

Syntax for truncation and wild cards will differ among platforms, so it is best to refer to the Help or Advanced Search section of the database platform website.

Proximity Operators

Proximity operators are a logic syntax that allow searchers to search words within certain proximity of each other. For example, *breast NEAR/2 cancer** in Embase will locate the root word of *cancer* within two words of *breast*. Kristensen found that applying proximity operators to locate words within the same sentence reduced recall by 74 percent and increased precision by 18 percent (Kristensen 1993). With the exception of PubMed Medline, most database platforms allow for proximity searching. The operators and syntax will vary among the database platforms and can be found in the Help or Advanced Search sections of most database platform websites.

Limits and Filters

Most databases provide ways to automatically limit searches by factors like tagging controlled vocabulary as a major focus, age of study participants, human, types of study, language, or publication date. Using such database-supplied limits affects the performance of a search. The most obvious reason is the time lapse between when a citation record is added to a database and when that record is updated with standard indexing which includes limits. Studies show that records are not always accurately or thoroughly indexed with database-supplied limits (Deacon, Smith, and Tow 2001; Funk and Reid 1983; Jenuwine and Floyd 2004). Restricting controlled vocabulary in Medline to only those citations where that concept is considered a major concept of the article has been shown to decrease recall by nearly 60 percent (Wright et al. 1991).

The best way to apply limits is to do so in such a way that the search includes records indexed by a desired limit without missing records that meet that same description but that were not indexed that way. This can be achieved by the careful use of the Boolean logic operator *NOT*. Sampson et al. explain this method using the human limit as an example.

> This results in the construction "not animal (not animal and human)," which is used to exclude animal studies that do not involve humans and animals, rather than limiting to the desired "humans"—a simpler construction but one that would exclude studies not tagged as either but that included relevant human evidence.

When the inclusion and exclusion criteria dictate a limit to specific types of studies, it is safer to use *NOT* to exclude the undesired types of publications (Tenopir and Evena Shu 1989). For example, if the review is to be limited to randomized controlled trials, instead of limiting the search to the database-supplied limit for randomized controlled trials, using *NOT* to specifically remove publication types like editorials, comments, and letters in conjunction with a sensitive filter for randomized controlled trials would increase the precision without significantly impacting the recall.

Filters are search strategies that have been designed to retrieve specific types of information from databases. When you design a search strategy for a systematic review, you are designing a search filter. Some filters have been tested and validated with reported precision and recall performance like the PubMed Clinical Queries filters (2015). Librarians can benefit from looking for previously constructed search filters to aid in the development of their own. However, caution should be taken when considering applying filters as part of designing a search strategy. Often search filters have been created and tested within a specific context, and if the context of the search you are designing is different, then it may not perform as effectively. Several studies show that when tested independently for reproducibility of performance, many filters do not perform well (Glanville, Kaunelis, and Mensinkai 2009; Golder and Loke 2012; Hempel et al. 2011; McKibbon, Wilczynski, and Haynes 2009; Yousefi-Nooraie et al. 2013). Furthermore, effectively adapting a previously constructed filter to the needs of a different research study requires an understanding of how filters are developed (Jenkins 2004). When a search filter is adapted, it is important to reference the original filter in notes and to include it in the written methods section regarding search development.

ADAPTATION ACROSS DATABASES

According to Sampson et al., errors in translating a search from one database to the next can significantly impact the precision and recall of that search (Sampson et al. 2008). All natural language terms used for one database platform search should be used in all database searches when it is feasible. An example where it may not be feasible occurs in PubMed because of the PubMed phrase index. In PubMed if you have a phrase in quotes and that phrase is not in the PubMed phrase index, PubMed will not search that phrase. It will also show an error "Quoted phrase not found" at the top of the page. PubMed will break the "Quoted phrase not found" into individual terms and apply automatic term matching to each one (Nahin 2003). Additionally, since PubMed does not allow for proximity searching, you will not be able to translate a proximity search into PubMed. The closest you can come is to AND terms in PubMed that you had searched with proximity operators in other database platforms. Doing this will greatly decrease the precision of the search.

The goal here is to translate a search you created from one database to operate as similarly as possible in the next database. This means that the controlled vocabulary, natural language terms, and all other field tags and operators used should be as similar as possible. For example, the proximity operator in Ovid Medline is *adj* and *NEAR/* in Embase, so *breast adj2 cancer* in Ovid Medline should be translated *breast NEAR/2 cancer* in Embase. If you have applied a field tag to a search term in one database, be sure to use the affiliated field tag and syntax in another database. For example, cancer limited to the title field, *cancer.ti.*, in Ovid Medline should be translated to *cancer:ti* in Cochrane Library. Note that even though the tags are the same, the platforms use different syntax. In Ovid Medline, the controlled vocabulary term for breast cancer is *exp Breast Neoplasms/* exploded or *Breast Neoplasms/* unexploded while in Cochrane Library the same controlled vocabulary term has different syntax *[mh "Breast Neoplasms"]* exploded or *[mh ^"Breast Neoplasms"]* unexploded. As you are adapting searches across databases, it may help to make a cheat sheet like the one in table 5.2.

Line vs. Paragraph Construction

The PRESS guideline emphasizes the importance of having a peer review a search for accuracy concerning whether line numbers have been combined with Boolean logic properly. In their very thorough systematic review of related literature they found no studies that discussed the issue of using wrong line numbers; however the researchers agreed that combining line numbers incorrectly could have a significant impact on search performance. They concluded that this was so self-evident that further study was unnecessary (Sampson et al. 2008). This conclusion reveals an assumption on the part of the researchers that everyone constructs searches in a line-by-line format. However, Bramer made an argument for constructing a search in one line or paragraph showing that doing so makes translation of keywords from one database to another easier, even enabling the use of macros in Word to do so automatically (Bramer 2014). Such an approach also makes saving all searches in a Word document possible as opposed to having to save the searches in each database platform for which users are required to log into their accounts. Furthermore, using paragraph searching makes reproducing the search by other users much easier since all they have to do is copy the search and paste it into the appropriate database. As of this writing, there are no studies comparing the two approaches. However, assuming that one performs better than the other is not self-evident and merits investigation.

ACTION BOX 5.1. USING PRESS TO EVALUATE A SEARCH STRATEGY

Find a systematic review in your discipline that reports at least one full search strategy. Before studying the search strategy, create a search strategy of your own on the topic. Then use the PRESS checklist to review the search, checking for mistakes. Also use PRESS on the search strategy reported in the article. Compare the searches. Did they make any mistakes? How does your search improve upon the one provided, and vice versa?

Table 5.2. Controlled vocabulary examples

Controlled vocabulary in . . .	*Exploded*	*Unexploded*	*Phrase*	*Unexploded phrase*	*Major focus*
Ovid Medline	exp Vaccines/	Vaccines/	exp Breast Neoplasms/	Breast Neoplasms/	exp *Breast Neoplasms/
Embase.com	'vaccine'/exp	'vaccine'/de	'breast cancer'/exp	'breast cancer'/de	'breast cancer'/exp/mj
EBSCO CINAHL	(MH "Vaccines+")	(MH "Vaccines")	(MH "Breast Neoplasms+")	(MH "Breast Neoplasms")	(MM "Breast Neoplasms+")
Wiley Cochrane	[mh vaccines]	[mh ^vaccines]	[mh "breast neoplasms"]	[mh ^"breast neoplasms"]	[mh "breast neoplasms" [mj]]
PubMed Medline	"Vaccines"[Mesh]	"Vaccines" [Mesh:NoExp]	"Breast Neoplasms"[Mesh]	"Breast Neoplasms" [Mesh:NoExp]	"Breast Neoplasms" [Majr]

CONCLUSION

Exhaustive systematic review literature searches require searching more than one resource. Resources to be searched should be chosen in a well-informed and deliberate way. Searchers should familiarize themselves with the content covered in each resource and available advanced searching tools. Librarians must design search strategies systematically and keep careful notes throughout the process.

REFERENCES

Booth, Andrew, Alan J. O'Rourke, and Nigel J. Ford. 2000. "Structuring the Presearch Reference Interview: A Useful Technique for Handling Clinical Questions." *Bulletin of the Medical Library Association* 88 (3): 239–46.

Bramer, Wichor. 2014. "Searching for Systematic Reviews: Set Numbers or One Liners?" *MLA News*, 1.

Deacon, Prue, Jill Buckley Smith, and Stephanie Tow. 2001. "Using Metadata to Create Navigation Paths in the HealthInsite Internet Gateway." *Health Information & Libraries Journal* 18 (1): 20–29.

Funk, Mark E., and Carolyn A. Reid. 1983. "Indexing Consistency in MEDLINE." *Bulletin of the Medical Library Association* 71 (2): 176.

Gavel, Y., and L. Iselid. 2008. "Web of Science and Scopus: A Journal Title Overlap Study." *Online Information Review* 32 (1): 8–21. doi:10.1108/14684520810865958.

Glanville, J., D. Kaunelis, and S. Mensinkai. 2009. "How Well Do Search Filters Perform in Identifying Economic Evaluations in MEDLINE and EMBASE." *International Journal of Technology Assessment in Health Care* 25 (4): 522–29. doi:10.1017/S0266462309990523.

Golder, S., and Y. K. Loke. 2012. "Sensitivity and Precision of Adverse Effects Search Filters in MEDLINE and EMBASE: A Case Study of Fractures with Thiazolidinediones." *Health Information and Libraries Journal* 29 (1): 28–38. doi:10.1111/j.1471-1842.2011.00972.x.

Haddaway, N. R., A. M. Collins, D. Coughlin, and S. Kirk. 2015. "The Role of Google Scholar in Evidence Reviews and Its Applicability to Grey Literature Searching." *PLoS One* 10 (9): e0138237. doi:10.1371/journal.pone.0138237.

Hausner, E., C. Guddat, T. Hermanns, U. Lampert, and S. Waffenschmidt. 2015. "Development of Search Strategies for Systematic Reviews: Validation Showed the Noninferiority of the Objective Approach." *Journal of Clinical Epidemiology* 68 (2): 191–99. doi:10.1016/j.jclinepi.2014.09.016.

Hausner, E., S. Waffenschmidt, T. Kaiser, and M. Simon. 2012. "Routine Development of Objectively Derived Search Strategies." *Systematic Reviews* no. 1:19. doi:10.1186/2046-4053-1-19.

Hempel, S., L. V. Rubenstein, R. M. Shanman, R. Foy, S. Golder, M. Danz, and P. G. Shekelle. 2011. "Identifying Quality Improvement Intervention Publications:

A Comparison of Electronic Search Strategies." *Implementation Science* 6 (1). doi:10.1186/1748-5908-6-85.

Higgins, Julian P. T., and Sally Green. 2011. *Cochrane Handbook for Systematic Reviews of Interventions*. http://handbook.cochrane.org.

Jenkins, M. 2004. "Evaluation of Methodological Search Filters—A Review." *Health Information and Libraries Journal* 21 (3): 148–63.

Jenuwine, Elizabeth S, and Judith A. Floyd. 2004. "Comparison of Medical Subject Headings and Text-Word Searches in MEDLINE to Retrieve Studies on Sleep in Healthy Individuals." *Journal of the Medical Library Association* 92 (3): 349.

Kristensen, Jaana. 1993. "Expanding End-Users' Query Statements for Free Text Searching with a Search-Aid Thesaurus." *Information Processing & Management* 29 (6): 733–44. doi:http://dx.doi.org/10.1016/0306-4573(93)90102-J.

McKibbon, K. A., N. L. Wilczynski, and R. B. Haynes. 2009. "Retrieving Randomized Controlled Trials from Medline: A Comparison of 38 Published Search Filters." *Health Information and Libraries Journal* 26 (3): 187–202. doi:10.1111/j.1471-1842.2008.00827.x.

Moher, D., A. Liberati, J. Tetzlaff, D. G. Altman, and the PRISMA Group. 2016. *PRISMA Transparent Reporting of Systematic Reviews and Meta-Analyses*. University of Oxford. http://www.prisma-statement.org.

Morton, Sally, Laura Levit, Alfred Berg, and Jill Eden. 2011. *Finding What Works in Health Care: Standards for Systematic Reviews*. Washington, DC: National Academies Press.

Nahin, A. M. 2003. "Change to PubMed's Automatic Term Mapping Affects Phrase Searching." *NLM Tech Bull*, no. 331:e3.

National Center for Biotechnology Information. 2015. "PubMed Help." Bethesda, MD: National Center for Biotechnology Information. http://www.ncbi.nlm.nih.gov/books/NBK3827.

Port, Toby. 1997. "PubMed: Basic Boolean Search Hints." *NLM Technical Bulletin*.

ProQuest. 2016. *ProQuest Dissertations & Theses Global*. ProQuest LLC. http://www.proquest.com/products-services/pqdtglobal.html.

Sampson, Margaret, Jessie McGowan, Elise Cogo, Jeremy Grimshaw, David Moher, and Carol Lefebvre. 2009. "An Evidence-Based Practice Guideline for the Peer Review of Electronic Search Strategies." *Journal of Clinical Epidemiology* 62 (9): 944–52. doi:http://dx.doi.org/10.1016/j.jclinepi.2008.10.012.

Sampson, Margaret, Jessie McGowan, Carol Lefebvre, David Moher, and J. M. Grimshaw. 2008. "PRESS: Peer Review of Electronic Search Strategies."

Silverman, E., S. Weiss, S. Shapiro, and D. Lomas. 2005. *Respiratory Genetics*. Boca Raton, FL: CRC Press.

Tenopir, Carol, and Man Evena Shu. 1989. "Magazines in Full Text: Uses and Search Strategies." *Online Review* 13 (2): 107–18.

U.S. National Library of Medicine. 2015a. *Fact Sheet Medical Subject Heading (MeSH)*. https://www.nlm.nih.gov/pubs/factsheets/mesh.html.

U.S. National Library of Medicine. 2015b. *Fact Sheet Medline*. U.S. National Library of Medicine. https://www.nlm.nih.gov/pubs/factsheets/medline.html.

Wiley. 2012. The Cochrane Library Reference Guide. http://www.cochranelibrary.com/dotAsset/5bc276c9-62ae-4ee2-987b-1641b4f753bb.pdf.

Wong, S. S., N. L. Wilczynski, and R. B. Haynes. 2004. "Developing optimal search strategies for detecting clinically relevant qualitative studies in MEDLINE." *Stud Health Technol Inform* no. 107 (Pt 1): 311–16.

Wright, L. C., H. J. Sutherland, J. I. Jackson, and J. E. Till. 1991. "Comparison of Search Strategies on CD Plus/MEDLINE." *CMAJ* 145 (5): 457–64.

Yousefi-Nooraie, R., S. Irani, S. Mortaz-Hedjri, and B. Shakiba. 2013. "Comparison of the Efficacy of Three PubMed Search Filters in Finding Randomized Controlled Trials to Answer Clinical Questions." *Journal of Evaluation in Clinical Practice* 19 (5): 723–26. doi:10.1111/j.1365-2753.2010.01554.x.

Chapter Six

Identifying the Studies, Part 2

Beyond Database Searching

Sarah T. Jewell, Susan Fowler,
and Margaret J. Foster

There's so much grey to every story—nothing is so black and white.

—Lisa Ling

OBJECTIVES

- Identify grey literature resources that should be searched
- Describe standards
- Identify additional search techniques
- List strategies to determine when to stop searching
- Describe techniques to evaluate the search
- After the screening, modifying the search

OVERVIEW

Databases of peer-reviewed journal articles are just one type of resource used to locate potential studies. Beyond database searching, there are a variety of other types of resources to search as well as other methods. Other sources include conference proceedings, research registries, clinical trials, dissertations and theses, reports from professional or organizational websites, and databases specifically designed to collect grey literature, or literature produced by organizations that are not traditional publishers. Other methods of searching include reference searching, hand searching, and advertising or requesting studies. This chapter will cover searching these other resources and using other search methods, as well as the standards for conducting, documenting, and reporting these options.

PUBLICATION BIAS

When searching for systematic reviews, if one wants to truly discover all that is out there, one cannot stop at searching major databases. The existence of publication bias necessitates that the search continue. Publication bias is when what appears in published literature is unrepresentative of all the completed research on the topic, thus potentially leading to the wrong conclusion. Publication bias can come from many angles, including outcome bias, where articles that show a significant result are more likely to be published; language bias, such as inclusion of only studies in English; availability bias, or inclusion of research that is readily available to the researcher; cost bias, or inclusion of only free or low-cost resources; and familiarity bias, or preference toward literature coming from one's own field of inquiry (Rothstein, Sutton, and Borenstein 2006). It is important that librarians make researchers aware of these biases, although it may not be practical in all cases to eliminate every one of them. At times, a researcher may be limited by language, not having the language skills or money to pay for translations, but in this case, the language bias should be acknowledged in the systematic review reporting.

What is the primary solution to eliminating publication bias? Grey literature is the solution, and its definition, according to the Fourth International Conference on Grey Literature, held in Washington, D.C., in October 1999, is "that which is produced on all levels of government, academics, business and industry in print and electronic formats, but which is not controlled by commercial publishers" (New York Academy of Medicine 2016).

LIBRARIAN'S CORNER 6.1

Q: What if my patrons argue that grey literature should not be included because it is not peer reviewed?

A: Tell them that the inclusion of grey literature in meta-analyses has been shown to change the results of whether interventions are considered effective or not (McAuley et al. 2000).

GREY LITERATURE

Conference Proceedings

Conference proceedings list abstracts for papers or posters presented at conferences. The information presented in these papers and posters may never

Table 6.1. Standards for searching beyond databases

Type of search	*MECIR*	*What Works*	*PRISMA*	*Document/report*
Research registers	Not mentioned			List grant or ID numbers of projects, in addition to principal investigator and title of project
Clinical trial registers	C27 mandatory	3.2.1	Item 7 Information Sources	List number of results and how many were selected from the set
Advertising/contacting	C31 highly desirable	3.2.2 and 3.2.3	Item 7 Information Sources	List names of groups contacted or how individuals were selected
Hand searching	Not mentioned	3.2.4	Item 7 Information Sources	List of resources and years searched. How it was searched (table of contents, page by page)
Citation searching	C29, C30 mandatory		Item 7 Information Sources	List which resources' references were screened
Grey literature -conference proceedings -dissertation/theses -Internet searching -government, IGO, NGOs	C28 mandatory	3.2.1 and 3.2.5		

be published in more traditional formats that are indexed with bibliographic control and thus easy to find, like research articles or book chapters. According to the Agency for Healthcare Research and Quality, "reviewers should routinely consider searching conference abstracts and proceedings to identify unpublished or unidentified studies" (Balshem et al. 2008). Hand searching conference proceedings is also a standard in guidelines provided by the National Academies and the Cochrane Collaboration (Higgins and Green 2011; Morton, Levit, Berg, and Eden 2011).

Locating some conference proceedings can be done via an electronic database search. Conference proceeding abstracts are often listed in journal supplement issues which may be indexed in citation databases like Medline, Embase, Scopus, the Cochrane Central Register of Controlled Trials, and Academic Search Premier. However, indexing of conference proceedings is not as broad as research articles. A thorough search of conference proceedings includes a hand search of supplement issues of on-topic journals and topic-appropriate association websites. Searching topic-appropriate association websites can be difficult for librarians. For example, a systematic review on a topic in pediatric emergency medicine should include a hand search of abstracts from the Advanced Pediatric Emergency Assembly from the past ten years (https://www.acep.org/pem/topics). Each assembly has its own website, and access requires membership in the American College of Emergency Physicians (ACEP). Since membership to the ACEP requires one to be an emergency medicine physician, librarians will be unable to search these conference sites (https://webapps.acep.org/MemberApp/AcepMemberApp.aspx). However, the librarian can guide topic experts of the review team to such sites.

Most conference abstracts will not be complete enough to include in a quantitative analysis of currently available evidence. However, conference abstracts will point to experts that can be contacted and to raw data that could impact results of an analysis.

Research Registries

There are several different types of research registries that range from those that keep individual participant data to registries that keep track of all the studies a particular organization has funded. There is even a register for systematic reviews called PROSPERO. What research registries to search depends on the central question a systematic review is attempting to answer. Searching and also using research registries to register research projects accomplishes three goals: reduction of duplicate studies and thus wasted effort, reduction of bias by providing transparency and comparison of study results to the original protocol, and reduction of publication bias by accessing study data not published in the more traditional research article.

The Breast Cancer Family Registry (Breast CFR) and the Colon Cancer Family Registry (Colon CFR), known collectively as Cancer Family Registries (CFRs), are examples of individual patient data research registries. The CFRs provide access to data like cancer-susceptible genes, biospecimens, and family histories (Epidemiology and Genomics Research Program 2015). Such registries are a must for individual patient data meta-analyses. Individual patient data meta-analyses are systematic reviews where, instead of analyzing the data reported in a research article, the researchers analyze and, when possible, quantify the raw individual patient data behind each published research article (Cochrane Collaboration 2016).

NIH RePORTER is a tool that allows searchers to find research projects funded by the National Institutes of Health (NIH) and any resulting publications and patents from those projects (Office of Extramural Research 2012). Searching NIH RePORTER can give systematic reviewers a fuller picture of any registered studies they are considering using in their review and also studies with data that may not appear anywhere else.

PROSPERO is an international systematic review registry. Systematic reviewers are supposed to register with PROSPERO at the inception of their project by reporting their study protocol. Searching PROSPERO can reduce duplication when researchers locate a systematic review in process that is attempting to answer the same question they are. Reviewing protocols for systematic reviews written by others can help researchers develop their own protocols. Comparing the protocol with the final reported outcomes helps reviewers assess the strength of methodology of a study and can even provide an opportunity for researchers to redo a systematic review using stronger methods.

Clinical Trials

One type of research registry is the clinical trial registry. As with research registries in general, the aim of clinical trial registries is to reduce publication bias and increase efficiency of medical research by reducing unnecessary study duplication. Several countries require clinical trials conducted in their countries or funded by their governments to be registered. For systematic reviewers, clinical trial registries provide information about studies that are in process which could affect the results of their systematic review once concluded and concluded studies with results that may not be published anywhere else. It is important to note that sometimes, even when reports of research have been published in an article, there may still be information about results in a registry that were not published in the article.

Requirements for who, what, and how clinical trials are registered differ across the world. The World Health Organization is currently attempting to gain consensus on reporting requirements and standards and to create a single entry point for all clinical trial registries (Karam, Kieny, Moorthy, and Vannice 2015). Currently, the search platform provided by the WHO, the International Clinical Trials Registry Platform (ICTRP), provides access to fifteen clinical trial registries, including clinicaltrials.gov. Clinicaltrials.gov is the most widely used and also oldest clinical trial registry available (U.S. National Library of Medicine 2015).

Dissertations/Theses

There is some evidence that theses and dissertations may not add much to a systematic review (Vickers and Smith 2000). However, this depends on the discipline and topic of the search. In cases where the topic is particularly new or research is scarce, sometimes one may find a dissertation on the subject before finding a more widely published article.

There are some ways that librarians can contribute to theses and dissertations being used as grey literature. First, they can help their institutions establish quality control of the theses shared, particularly with respect to what version of the thesis is posted. Second, librarians can help select the metadata standard that will be used in the institutional repository and assist with the cataloging of these records. Third, ideally the full text of dissertations should be made available in a standard format, depending on the nature of the discipline. While MS Word documents and PDFs seem standard, in some fields it may make more sense for the records to be in XML or LaTeX format. Fourth, by selecting a standard format for deposit, exchange, and harvesting (e.g., OAI-PMH), the librarians involved can increase the interoperability of the theses database in question, and at the same time increase the discoverability of the theses. Finally, offering services along with access to the institutional repository allows the librarians to fulfill the needs of the users of the repositories. Services can include discussion of theses via social media, usage statistics and metrics, print-on-demand services, and preservation (Schopfel 2013).

Google Site Search of Professional Organization Websites

Another type of grey literature that can be located by searching nontraditional sources is to locate white papers and reports available on the websites of professional, government, business, and nonprofit organizations. Although these reports may not be peer reviewed, they are important to include due to the biases inherent in scholarly publishing. White papers or reports can be

Table 6.2. Sources for theses and dissertations

Database	*URL*	*Description*
Open Access Theses and Dissertations	https://oatd.org	An index of over 2.4 million electronic theses and dissertations
ProQuest Theses & Dissertations		Subscription database
British Library EThOS (Electronic Theses Online Service)	http://EThOS.bl.uk	
TROVE Australian theses	http://trove.nla.gov.au/general/theses	

produced in a timelier manner than peer-reviewed publications and may help to alleviate outcome bias and other related biases.

One trick to locate these reports that may be somewhat hidden in these websites is to utilize Google's site search feature (e.g., *site:ons.org*). Google's deep indexing allows for searching of websites using keyword searches. The systematic review search often must be simplified, as the search string is generally limited to thirty-two words, but this can be done by prioritizing the keywords and also by eliminating concept categories that are a given for the organization in question. For example, if one is searching for articles on interrater reliability among dermatologists for the diagnosis of skin cancer, if you are searching the website of the American Academy of Dermatology, you might be able to eliminate the concept of dermatologist in the search, since the majority of the documents on the website will be related to dermatology regardless. Another limitation of doing this type of search is that many results, often too numerous to review, are generated. A way to limit this is to prespecify the number of top records that will be reviewed (e.g., the top twenty retrieved) and record how many are reviewed and how many among those are relevant. Some will argue that Google searches are not truly replicable, due to complicated ranking algorithms, which at times even bias the searcher toward results that may be more popular in his or her geographical location, but the potential value of the reports found may, at times, outweigh these concerns.

Grey Literature Databases

Searching for grey literature in repositories specifically designed to capture grey literature is another method to broaden the search. Like the Google site searches, it is not always possible to search the full detailed search strategy

Table 6.3. Grey literature databases

Database	*URL*	*Fields included*
OpenDOAR	http://opendoar.org	Directory of academic repositories
GreyLit.org	http://greylit.org (no longer updated as of January 2017)	Medicine, prioritizing the areas of prevention, healthy aging, disparities, and history of medicine
Open Grey	http://www.opengrey.eu	European documents on science, technology, biomedical science, economics, social science, and humanities

in these repositories, but modified, usually simplified searches must be done instead.

Government and International Organizations

Once, government documents were hard to find, having to be retrieved by document number in a physical library. Now, many governments offer more readily accessible documents one can find on the web.

Table 6.4. Government and international databases

Government database	*URL*	*Fields included*
Northwestern University LibGuide on International Resources by Theme	http://libguides.northwestern.edu/international	Agriculture, crime and drugs, economics, education, finance, etc.
World Health Organization	http://www.who.it	International health publications and data from within the United Nations
Organisation for Economic Co-operation and Development (OECD) iLibrary	http://www.oecd-ilibrary.org	Documents on policies that affect social and economic well-being around the world
Science.gov	https://www.science.gov	U.S. government science documents
World Bank Open Data	http://data.worldbank.org	Open access data to global development data
International Monetary Fund	http://www.imf.org	IMF is an organization of 189 countries; reports and data sets

OTHER TYPES OF SEARCHING

Hand Searching

Hand searching is a term used to describe browsing resources to find relevant studies. There are several reasons for doing this. First, some journals are not well indexed. For example, *Bovine Practitioner* is a well-known journal in cattle health; however, it is not indexed in Medline, and the conference abstracts are not indexed in CAB Abstracts, two of the most frequently searched databases for veterinary medicine. Secondly, some parts of journals are not indexed, such as conference abstracts and supplements. Lastly, many resources are not indexed in any database and can only be browsed. To select resources to hand search, one must know a great deal about the particular subject area to know what journals, conference proceedings, or other resources need to be searched which are not covered well by commercially or publically available databases. While some have questioned the value of hand searching and this form of searching was removed from Methodological Expectations of Cochrane Intervention Reviews (MECIR), others continue to advocate for its use. Hopewell wrote that hand searching was most useful in "identifying trials reported as abstracts, letters and those published in languages other than English, together with all reports published in journals not indexed in electronic databases." They did however conclude that if time is limited, a well-developed search would retrieve the majority of English-language study reports (if most of the topic-specific relevant journals are indexed by the database) (Hopewell et al. 2007).

Cited Reference Searching

Reviewing references cited by included and highly relevant articles such as related reviews is an important step in finding potentially eligible studies. This is important because it can identify articles that were not indexed in already searched databases, locate articles that did not use commonly used keywords, or highlight grey literature that these articles cited. In addition, resources that have cited the included and relevant articles could also be screened. While searching for citing articles of included articles is not standard, it is a logical step to find potential articles. Methods for conducting the search for cited and citing references include: browsing the references at the end of each article (will only show the cited references) or using a citation tracking database (Scopus, Web of Science, Google Scholar) to locate both cited and citing references. Documentation of this process should cover which articles references/citing articles were screened and what resources were used to find them (if any). Of course, this process cannot be conducted until the articles retrieved from database searches and other search approaches are completed and the articles screened (as discussed in chapter 8).

Advertising for Studies/Contacting Potential Study Authors

Requesting studies is a way to solicit studies that were not published, are about to be published, were published in harder-to-find journals, and so on. Authors should first determine methods to contact potential study authors such as professional organizations, listservs, or directly to known authors. Authors should document how they reached out to find studies.

NEXT STEPS IN THE SEARCH PROCESS

After the Search

If, after utilizing techniques of searching beyond the database searches, additional studies are identified from these efforts, the librarian should determine if these articles are indexed in the databases that were searched first. If so, there may be keywords that were missed in the original database searches, and other relevant articles may have also been missed. Box 6.1 demonstrates a technique for determining the terms that may have been missed.

Evaluation of the Search

Calculating the precision of a search is one way to evaluate a search strategy. Precision is represented by the number of relevant records retrieved as a proportion of the total number of records retrieved (Jenkins and Johnson 2004).

When to Stop Searching

One question often asked of review authors when meeting an information specialist is "when do I stop searching?" There are several issues to consider when answering this question. First is the issue of currency, with some journals requiring that a search be updated within six months of publication. This may mean that after a study has been accepted for publication, the search needs to be updated. By setting up alerts and saving the searches in the native databases in the beginning, sometimes this can speed up the process of updating the search. Besides the need for transparent and clear methods, well-documented search processes will assist in updating the searches efficiently. How updated does the search need to be? Often when updating the searches, only a select few databases, usually the primary ones which retrieved the highest number of relevant records, need to be searched.

ACTION BOX 6.1. DETERMINING WHY AN ARTICLE WAS NOT RETRIEVED IN A SEARCH

Scenario: Articles 1 and 2 and 3 are selected to be included after searching grey literature resources. In reviewing these articles, these three were indexed in Medline. Article 2 was not retrieved during the original search because of the date the search was run; it was found when rerunning the search. Article 3 was not indexed in Medline. To determine why article 1 does not appear, the following steps are taken.

First, break your search into components where the ANDs are happening, especially if you designed the search in paragraph form. The table below shows a search with three components and its synonyms.

Component	*Original search (synonyms for each concept)*	*Test article*	*results*
Concept A	a1 or a2 or a3 or a4	(terms for concept A) and article	1 result—it is in this group
Concept B	b1 or b2 or b3 or b4	(terms for concept B) and article	0 results—It Is due to this concept that the article did not appear
Concept C	c1 or c2 or c3 or c4	(terms for concept B) and article	1 result—it is in this group

Now that you know it was concept B that was lacking for article 1, you will need to find a term matching it in the title, abstract, or thesaurus/index terms. You will then retrieve new articles after de-duplicating it with the old search to see what new records are retrieved.

Second is the issue of thoroughness. Is the search complete? Have all the resources selected to search been searched? Were new resources found in the last search? In order to inform when one might stop a systematic search, one can use the capture-mark-recapture (CMR) method which is derived from ecological population studies. This method is modeled after the technique of capturing animals, marking them, releasing them back into the wild, and then recording how often they are recaptured. The number of animals (or in the case of a systematic review, studies) that are recaptured can be used to estimate the population size. The steps of the CMR are as follows: (1) define an estimation of completeness for the systematic review, such as a percentage of articles and saturation; (2) perform the search in the databases expected to produce the highest number of relevant studies and screen for final inclusion; (3) calculate the horizon estimate, or population estimate; (4) compare retrieval with the horizon estimate to see if the completeness criteria were met; (5) continue searching additional sources until an estimate of completeness is satisfied (Lane et al. 2013).

In addition to the CMR method, Cooper recommends some questions to consider when deciding whether or not to stop searching: (1) Have you searched all the databases likely to contain the highest numbers of relevant citations? (2) Have you verified that there are no major biases of omission, such as excluding non-English sources? (3) Have you modified your search strategy by adding terms based on citations highly relevant to your topic? (4) How many new unique and relevant citations did you add to the latest two versions of your search? (5) When you compare complementary databases, how many new, unique, and relevant citations have you discovered in the last two searches? (6) If you conducted author searches on the three or four most prolific authors on your topic, can you identify any new relevant citations on your topic (Cooper, Hedges, and Valentine 2009)?

CONCLUSION

It is important to search beyond peer-reviewed bibliographic databases to ensure that all eligible studies are located. While there are controversies over the usefulness of these additional searches, Cochrane and other organizations continue to call for these searches in their standards.

REFERENCES

Balshem, H., A. Stevens, M. Ansari, S. Norris, D. Kansagara, T. Shamliyan, et al. 2008. "Finding Grey Literature Evidence and Assessing for Outcome and Analysis Reporting Biases When Comparing Medical Interventions: AHRQ and the Effective Health Care Program." *Methods Guide for Effectiveness and Comparative Effectiveness Reviews*.

Cochrane Collaboration. 2016. "About IPD Meta-Analyses." Retrieved from http://methods.cochrane.org/ipdma/about-ipd-meta-analyses.

Cooper, Harris M., Larry V. Hedges, and Jeff C. Valentine. 2009. *The Handbook of Research Synthesis and Meta-Analysis*. New York: Russell Sage Foundation.

Epidemiology and Genomics Research Program. 2015. Breast and Colon Cancer Family Registries. Retrieved from http://epi.grants.cancer.gov/CFR.

Higgins, Julian P. T., Sally Green, and Cochrane Collaboration. 2011. *Cochrane Handbook for Systematic Reviews of Interventions*. Chichester, England; Hoboken, NJ: Wiley-Blackwell.

Hopewell, S., S. McDonald, M. Clarke, and M. Egger. 2007. "Grey Literature in Meta-Analyses of Randomized Trials of Health Care Interventions." *The Cochrane Database of Systematic Reviews*.

Jenkins, M., and F. Johnson. 2004. "Awareness, Use and Opinions of Methodological Search Filters Used for the Retrieval of Evidence-Based Medical Literature—A Questionnaire Survey." *Health Information and Libraries Journal* 21 (1): 33–43.

Karam, Ghassan, Marie-Paule Kieny, Vasee S. Moorthy, and Kirsten S. Vannice. 2015. "Rationale for WHO's New Position Calling for Prompt Reporting and Public Disclosure of Interventional Clinical Trial Results." *PLOS Medicine* 12(4): e1001819.doi:10.1371/journal.pmed.1001819.

Lane, D., J. Dykeman, M. Ferri, C. H. Goldsmith, and H. T. Stelfox. 2013. "Capture-Mark-Recapture as a Tool for Estimating the Number of Articles Available for Systematic Reviews in Critical Care Medicine." *Journal of Critical Care* 28 (4): 469–75.

McAuley, Laura, et al. 2000. "Does the Inclusion of Grey Literature Influence Estimates of Intervention Effectiveness Reported in Meta-Analyses?" *Lancet* 356 (9237): 1228.

Morton, Sally, Laura Levit, Alfred Berg, and Jill Eden. 2011. *Finding What Works in Health Care: Standards for Systematic Reviews*. Washington, DC: National Academies Press.

New York Academy of Medicine. 2016. "What Is Grey Literature?" http://www.greylit.org/about.

Office of Extramural Research. 2012. "RePORTER Frequently Asked Questions (FAQs)." https://report.nih.gov/faq.aspx?sid=2#36.

Rothstein, H. R., A. J. Sutton, and M. Borenstein. 2006. "Publication Bias in Meta-Analysis: Prevention, Assessment and Adjustments." In *Publication Bias in Meta-Analysis: Prevention, Assessment and Adjustments*, 1–356. Chichester, England; Hoboken, NJ: Wiley, 2005.

Schopfel, J. 2013. "Adding Value to Electronic Theses and Dissertations in Institutional Repositories." *D-Lib Magazine* 19 (3–4).

U.S. National Library of Medicine. 2015. "ClinicalTrials.gov Background." https://clinicaltrials.gov/ct2/about-site/background.

Vickers, A. J., and C. Smith. 2000. "Research Note: Incorporating Data from Dissertations in Systematic Reviews." *International Journal of Technology Assessment in Health Care* 16 (2): 711–13.

Chapter Seven

Identifying the Studies, Part 3

Case Studies

Margaret J. Foster, Sarah T. Jewell,
and Guest Authors

An expert is a man who has made all the mistakes which can be made, in a narrow field.

—Niels Bohr

OBJECTIVES

- To provide detailed examples of systematic review questions and eligibility criteria
- To demonstrate examples of systematic review searches of databases and grey literature

OVERVIEW

The search methods for systematic reviews form the starting point for data gathering and need to be well conducted and transparently reported. Attending workshops and training on systematic reviews and reading guides will only serve to introduce the skills needed to perform review searches. To improve expertise in searching for reviews will require a great deal of practice. As Niels Bohr said, making mistakes is part of the process, especially if one learns from the errors. By developing searches and having these peer reviewed, librarians can continue to improve their searching skills. Even those that have excellent searching skills can benefit from peer review, as other perspectives on the search can provide valuable feedback. Other ways to develop include seeking mentorship and shadowing someone's systematic review service. To this end, this chapter provides nine example review projects with searches developed by librarians across the disciplines.

Each of the following case studies focuses on a type of question within a specific discipline. The frameworks of the review questions were varied to demonstrate the variety of frameworks as presented in chapter 3 (see boxes 3.4 and 3.5). The selected bibliographic databases, grey literature sources, and details of additional types of searches are provided as examples of the suggestions provided in chapters 5 and 6. These searches are not meant to be perfect searches but instead a glimpse into searches that librarians conducted given a particular question. In addition, resources related to the field in question used in the case study are provided for further reading.

CASE STUDY 1: EFFECTIVENESS OF INTERVENTIONS IN THE FIELD OF VETERINARY MEDICINE

Heather K. Moberly and Margaret J. Foster

Planning

Question: What are the effectiveness of NSAIDS for dogs with osteoarthritis?
Framework: This question can be framed with the PICO format as detailed in box 7.1 (Richardson et al. 1995).

TEXTBOX 7.1. FRAMEWORK FOR CASE STUDY 1

P (population): dogs with osteoarthritis
I (intervention): NSAIDS
C (comparison): no medication
O (outcome): clinical signs

Identifying

Concepts searched: [dogs] and [NSAIDs] and [osteoarthritis]
Bibliographic Databases:
PubMed
(Antiinflammator* OR nsaid* OR nsaid OR antirheumatic* OR antirheumatic OR aspirin OR aspirin* OR carprofen OR carprofen* OR deracoxib

OR deracoxib* OR firocoxib OR firocoxib* OR galliprant OR galliprant* OR meloxicam OR meloxicam* OR etodolac OR etodolac* OR ketoprofen OR ketoprofen* OR naproxen OR naproxen* OR piroxicam OR piroxicam* OR tepoxalin OR tepoxalin*) AND (dogs OR dog OR dog diseases OR canine*) AND (Osteoarth* OR osteoarthritis OR DJD OR "Degenerative Joint Disease")

Cab abstracts (Ovid)

1. exp dogs/
2. (dog or dogs or canine or canines).mp.
3. or/1–2
4. exp non-steroidal antiinflammatory agents/
5. (nsaid* or antiinflammator* or antirheumatic* or antiinflammatory or antirheumatic or aspirin* or exp asprin or aspirin or carprofen or carprofen* or deracoxib or deracoxib* or firocoxib or firocoxib* or meloxicam or meloxicam* or etodolac or etodolac* or ketoprofen or ketoprofen* or exp ketoprofen or naproxen or naproxen* or piroxicam or piroxicam* or tepoxalin or tepoxalin*).mp.
6. or/4–5
7. exp osteoarthritis/
8. (osteoarth* or djd or degenerative joint disease).mp.
9. or/7–8
10. 3 and 6 and 9

Grey Literature:

- Searchable Proceedings of Animal Conferences (S-PAC)
  Link: https://spac.adsa.org
- Clinician's Brief
  Link: http://www.cliniciansbrief.com, unidexed journal, requires free login
- VetSRev: Database of veterinary systematic reviews
  Link: http://webapps.nottinghan.ac.uk/refbase
- International Veterinary Information Service (IVIS)
  Link: http://www.ivis.org, requires a free login
- American Academy of Veterinary Pharmacology and Therapeutics
  Link: http://www.aavpt.org

Related Resources/References

Centre for Evidence-based Veterinary Medicine (CEVM) http://www.nottingham.ac.uk/cevm/. Evidence Based Veterinary Medicine Association (EBVMA) https://ebvma.org/. Evidence Based Veterinary Network http://knowledge.rcvs.org.uk/evidence-based-veterinary-medicine/.

Grindlay, D. J. C., M. L. Brennan, and R. S. Dean. 2012. "Searching the veterinary literature: A comparison of coverage of veterinary journals by nine bibliographic

databases." *Journal of Veterinary Medical Education* 39 (4): 404–412. doi:10.3138/jvme.1111.109R.
Holmes, M. A. 2012. "Systematic reviews in small animal veterinary medicine: What they are and why do we need them?" *Journal of Small Animal Practice* 53 (4) 195–196. doi:10.1111/j.1748-5827.2011.01194.x.
O'Connor, A., and J. Sargeant. 2015. "Research synthesis in veterinary science: Narrative reviews, systematic reviews, and meta-analysis." *Veterinary Journal* 206: 261–267. doi:10.1016/j/tvjl.2015.08.025.
Systematic Reviews and Meta-Analysis in Animal Agriculture and Veterinary Medicine (Special Issue) Zoonoses and Public Health, 2014, volume 61 supplement 1. http://onlinelibrary.wiley.com/doi/10.1111/zph.2014.61.issue-S1/issuetoc. The supplement contains six open access articles covering the systematic review process from a veterinary perspective.
Systematic Reviews for Animals & Food (SYREAF) Education Section, Collection of articles written by SYREAF http://www.syreaf.org/education.
Waddell, L., A. Rajić, J. Sargeant, S. Parker, A. Deckert, and S. McEwen. 2009. "The Methodological Soundness of Literature Reviews Addressing Three Potential Zoonotic Public Health Issues." *Zoonoses and Public Health* 56 (9–10): 477–89. doi:10.1111/j.1863-2378.2008.01194.x.

CASE STUDY 2: PREVALENCE QUESTION IN THE FIELD OF DENTISTRY

Elizabeth Stellrecht

Planning

Question: What is the prevalence of periodontal disease in pregnant women, and what possible outcomes or risks may occur when both conditions are present?
Framework: This question can be framed with the PEO (population, exposure, outcome) framework, detailed in box 7.2 (Kahn et al. 2003).

TEXTBOX 7.2. FRAMEWORK FOR CASE STUDY 2

P (population): pregnant women
E (exposure): periodontal disease
O (outcome): potential risks

Identifying

Concepts searched: [Periodontal disease] AND [pregnant] AND [complications]

Bibliographic Databases:

PubMed

(((((“Pregnant Women”[Mesh]) OR “Pregnancy”[Mesh]) OR “pregnant women”)) AND (((((((((“Periodontal Diseases”[Mesh]) OR alveolar bone loss) OR gingivitis) OR periodon*) OR gingival bleeding) OR clinical attachment loss) OR periodontal attachment loss) OR periodontal pocket) OR pocket depth)) AND (((((((“Pregnancy Complications”[Mesh]) OR adverse pregnancy outcomes) OR pre eclampsia) OR low birth weight) OR gestational diabetes) OR premature birth) OR pregnancy induced hypertension)

Embase (Elsevier interface)

((‘pregnant women’/exp OR ‘pregnant women’) OR (‘pregnancy’/exp OR ‘pregnancy’)) AND ((‘periodontal diseases’/exp OR ‘periodontal diseases’) OR (‘alveolar bone loss’/exp OR ‘alveolar bone loss’) OR (‘gingivitis’/exp OR ‘gingivitis’) OR periodon* OR (‘gingival bleeding’/exp OR ‘gingival bleeding’) OR ‘clinical attachment loss’ OR (periodontal AND attachment AND loss) OR (‘periodontal pocket’/exp OR ‘periodontal pocket’) OR (pocket AND depth)) AND ((‘pregnancy complications’/exp OR ‘pregnancy complications’) OR (adverse AND (‘pregnancy’/exp OR pregnancy) AND outcomes) OR (‘pre eclampsia’/exp OR ‘pre eclampsia’) OR (‘low birth weight’/exp OR ‘low birth weight’) OR (‘gestational diabetes’/exp OR ‘gestational diabetes’) OR (‘premature birth’/exp OR ‘premature birth’) OR (‘pregnancy induced hypertension’/exp OR ‘pregnancy induced hypertension’))

Note: Term in quotes with/exp indicates an Emtree term, Embase’s subject heading language.

Evidence-Based Medicine Reviews (Cochrane Database)

((pregnancy.mp.) OR (Pregnant women.mp.)) AND (((((((((periodontal disease*.mp.) OR (alveolar bone loss.mp.) OR (gingivitis.mp.) OR (gingiva* bleeding.mp.) OR (periodon*.mp.) OR (clinical attachment loss.mp.) OR (periodontal attachment loss.mp.) OR (periodontal pocket*.mp.) OR (pocket depth.mp.)) AND (((((((pregnancy complication*.mp.) OR (adverse pregnancy outcome*.mp.) OR (pre eclampsia.mp.) OR (low birth weight.mp.) OR (gestational diabetes.mp.) OR (premature birth.mp.) OR (pregnancy induced hypertension.mp.))

CINAHL (EBSCO)

(((MH “Pregnancy+”) OR (MH “Expectant Mothers”) OR (“pregnant women”)) AND (((((((((MH “Periodontal Diseases+”) OR (alveolar bone loss) OR (MH “Gingivitis+”) OR (MH “Periodontal Attachment Loss”) OR (clinical attachment loss) OR (periodon*) OR (gingival bleeding) OR (MH "Periodontal Pocket") OR (pocket depth)) AND (((((((MH "Pregnancy Complications+") OR (adverse pregnancy outcomes) OR (MH "Pre-Eclampsia+") OR (MH "Infant, Low Birth Weight+") OR (MH "Diabetes Mellitus, Gestational") OR (MH "Childbirth, Premature") OR (MH "Pregnancy-Induced Hypertension+"))

Grey Literature:

- Grey literature databases: http://greylit.org (no longer updated as of January 2017) and http://opengrey.eu
- American Academy of Periodontics proceedings
  Link: https://www.perio.org/consumer/periodontal-regeneration-workshop-proceedings
- Clinicaltrials.gov

Hand Searching:

- *The Journal of Periodontology*

Related Resources

Standards, guides, or organizations related to the topic/discipline area:
At this time, there are no standards recommended by the American Dental Association (ADA) when writing a systematic review for dental medicine. Most journals in the dental literature require or recommend using the *Cochrane Collaboration Handbook* for conducting the review and the PRISMA statement for reporting.

The following organizations are dedicated to fostering evidence-based dentistry by leveraging the power of systematic reviews as well as creating evidence-based guidelines:

- The American Dental Association's Center for Evidence-Based Dentistry (http://ebd.ada.org/en). In addition to compiling dental medicine systematic reviews and guidelines, it also contains critical summaries of systematic reviews that summarize and critically appraise a systematic review.
- Centre for Evidence-Based Dentistry (http://www.cebd.org)
- Cochrane Oral Health Group (http://ohg.cochrane.org)

References important to dental systematic reviews:
The *Journal of the American Dental Association* recently published a series titled *The Journal of the American Dental Association Evidence-Based Practice Series*, many of which inform the researcher on how to critically appraise different types of study designs. These articles will be useful to individuals new to conducting systematic reviews.

Brignardello-Petersen, Romina, Alonso Carrasco-Labra, H. Austin Booth, Michael Glick, Gordon H. Guyatt, Amir Azarpazhooh, and Thomas Agoritsas. 2014. "A

Practical Approach to Evidence-Based Dentistry: How to Search for Evidence to Inform Clinical Decisions." *Journal of the American Dental Association (1939)* 145 (12): 1262–67. doi:10.14219/jada.2014.113.

Brignardello-Petersen, Romina, Alonso Carrasco-Labra, Michael Glick, Gordon H. Guyatt, and Amir Azarpazhooh. 2014. "A Practical Approach to Evidence-Based Dentistry: Understanding and Applying the Principles of EBD." *Journal of the American Dental Association (1939)* 145 (11): 1105–07. doi:10.14219/jada.2014.102.

———. 2015. "A Practical Approach to Evidence-Based Dentistry: III: How to Appraise and Use an Article about Therapy." *Journal of the American Dental Association (1939)* 146 (1): 49.e1. doi:10.1016/j.adaj.2014.11.010.

———. 2015. "A Practical Approach to Evidence-Based Dentistry: IV: How to Use an Article about Harm." *Journal of the American Dental Association (1939)* 146 (2): 101.e1. doi:10.1016/j.adaj.2014.12.002.

———. 2015. "A Practical Approach to Evidence-Based Dentistry: V: How to Appraise and Use an Article about Diagnosis." *Journal of the American Dental Association (1939)* 146 (3): 191.e1. doi:10.1016/j.adaj.2015.01.011.

Carrasco-Labra, Alonso, Romina Brignardello-Petersen, Michael Glick, Gordon H. Guyatt, and Amir Azarpazhooh. 2015. "A Practical Approach to Evidence-Based Dentistry: VI: How to Use a Systematic Review." *Journal of the American Dental Association (1939)* 146 (4): 265.e1. doi:10.1016/j.adaj.2015.01.025.

Sale, Joanna E. M., Maryam Amin, Alonso Carrasco-Labra, Romina Brignardello-Petersen, Michael Glick, Gordon H. Guyatt, and Amir Azarpazhooh. 2015. "A Practical Approach to Evidence-Based Dentistry: VIII: How to Appraise an Article Based on a Qualitative Study." *Journal of the American Dental Association (1939)* 146 (8): 623–30. doi:10.1016/j.adaj.2015.06.010.

CASE STUDY 3: QUALITY OF EXPERIENCE QUESTION IN THE FIELD OF NURSING

Margaret J. Foster

Planning

Question: What is the quality of life and lived experience of adult diabetic patients with foot ulcers?

Framework: This question can be framed with the SPIDER (sample, phenomenon of interest, design, evaluation, research type) framework designed for qualitative questions, as shown in box 7.3 (Cooke, Smith, and Booth 2012).

TEXTBOX 7.3. FRAMEWORK FOR CASE STUDY 3

S (sample): diabetic patients
PI (phenomenon of interest): dealing with foot ulcers
D (design): interviews or focus types
E (evaluation): experiences
R (research type): qualitative

Identifying

Concepts searched: [diabetes] and [foot ulcers] and [quality of life or lived experience]

Bibliographic Databases:

Medline (Ovid)

1. exp Diabetic Foot/
2. (diabet* adj3 (ulcer or feet or foot or wound* or amputat*)).ti,ab,kw.
3. (exp Diabetes Mellitus/ or diabet*.ti,ab,kw.) and exp Foot Ulcer/
4. or/1–3
5. exp "Quality of Life"/
6. exp Qualitative Research/ or exp Interviews as Topic/
7. ("lived experience" or "quality of life").ti,ab.
8. (patient adj3 (perspective* or experience* or attitude*)).ti,ab.
9. or/5–8
10. 4 and 9

CINAHL (EBSCO)

(MM "Diabetic Foot" OR TI (diabet* w3 (ulcer or feet or foot or wound* or amputat*)) OR AB (diabet* w3 (ulcer or feet or foot or wound* or amputat*))) AND ((MH "Diabetic Patients" or MH "Diabetes Mellitus+") OR TI diabet* OR AB diabet*) AND ((MH "Quality of Life+") OR AB ("quality of life" or qol or ((lived or life) w2 experience*) or (patient w3 (perspective* or experience* or attitude*))) or TI ("quality of life" or qol or ((lived or life) w2 experience*) or (patient w3 (perspective* or experience* or attitude*)))

Embase (Ovid)

1. exp Diabetic Foot/
2. (diabet* adj3 (ulcer or feet or foot or wound* or amputat*)).ti,ab,kw.
3. (exp Diabetes Mellitus/ or diabet*.ti,ab,kw.) and exp Foot Ulcer/
4. or/1–3

5. exp "Quality of Life"/ or exp personal experience/
6. exp Qualitative Research/ or exp Interviews as Topic/
7. ("lived experience" or "quality of life").ti,ab.
8. (patient adj3 (perspective* or experience* or attitude*)).ti,ab.
9. or/5–8
10. 4 and 9

PsycINFO (EBSCO)

((DE "Diabetes" OR DE "Diabetes Mellitus" OR DE "Gestational Diabetes" OR DE "Type 2 Diabetes") OR TI diabet* OR AB diabet*) AND TI ((foot or feet)) OR AB ((foot or feet))) OR TI (diabet* w3 (ulcer or feet or foot or wound* or amputat*)) OR AB (diabet* w3 (ulcer or feet or foot or wound* or amputat*))) AND ((DE "Life Experiences" OR DE "Life Changes") OR (DE "Quality of Life" OR DE "Quality of Work Life")) OR TI (("quality of life" or qol or ((lived or life) w2 experience*) or (patient w3 (perspective* or experience* or attitude*))) OR AB (("quality of life" or qol or ((lived or life) w2 experience*) or (patient w3 (perspective* or experience* or attitude*)))

Browse and/or request studies from following organizations:

- International Diabetes Federation: www.idf.org
- American Diabetes Association: www.diabetes.org
- American Association of Diabetes Educators: www.diabeteseducator.org
- American Podiatric Medical Association: www.apma.org
- Diabetes Care and Education: www.dce.org
- American Association of Clinical Endocrinologists: www.aace.com
- American Orthopaedic Foot and Ankle Society: http://www.aofas.org

Related Resources

Reviews related to this topic:

Albuquerque, de Almeida, Adriano Menis Ferreira, Maria Lucia Ivo, Marcelo Alessandro Rigotti, Regina Queiroz Gonçalves, and Santos Pereira Pelegrini dos. 2014. "Socio-Demographic and Clinic Characteristics and Quality of Life of People with Wounds: An Integrative Review." *Journal of Nursing UFPE/Revista De Enfermagem UFPE* 8 (12): 4361 9p.

Herber, Oliver R., Wilfried Schnepp, and Monika A. Rieger. 2007. "A Systematic Review on the Impact of Leg Ulceration on Patients' Quality of Life." *Health & Quality of Life Outcomes* 5:44.

Kossioris, Aristomenis, and T. Karousi. 2015. "Determinants of Health-Related Quality of Life in Patients with Diabetic Foot Ulcers: A Systematic Review and Meta-Analysis." *Health Science Journal* 9 (6): 7 7p.

van Acker, Kristien, Philippe Léger, Agnes Hartemann, Abhineet Chawla, and Mohd Kashif Siddiqui. 2014. "Burden of Diabetic Foot Disorders, Guidelines for Management and Disparities in Implementation in Europe: A Systematic Literature Review." *Diabetes/Metabolism Research & Reviews* 30 (8): 645 11p.

Nursing systematic reviews:

Bellali, Thalia. 2011. "The Basic Principles and Methodology of Quantitative Systematic Reviews." *Nosileftiki* 50 (1): 22 13p.
Butler, Ashleigh, Helen Hall, and Beverley Copnell. 2016. "A Guide to Writing a Qualitative Systematic Review Protocol to Enhance Evidence-Based Practice in Nursing and Health Care." *Worldviews on Evidence-Based Nursing* 13 (3): 249 9p.
Holopainen, A., T. Hakulinen-Viitanen, and K. Tossavainen. 2008. "Systematic Review—A Method for Nursing Research." *Nurse Researcher* 16 (1): 83 12p.
Jutel, Annemarie. 2012. "Method or Madness? The Dominance of the Systematic Review in Nursing Scholarship." *Aporia* 4 (4): 57 6p.
McCrae, Niall, Marlene Blackstock, and Edward Purssell. 2015. "Eligibility Criteria in Systematic Reviews: A Methodological Review." *International Journal of Nursing Studies* 52 (7): 1276 8p.
Pölkki, Tarja, Outi Kanste, Maria Kääriäinen, Satu Elo, and Helvi Kyngäs. 2014. "The Methodological Quality of Systematic Reviews Published in High-Impact Nursing Journals: A Review of the Literature." *Journal of Clinical Nursing* 23 (3): 332 18p.

CASE STUDY 4: THEORY RELATED QUESTION IN THE FIELD OF HEALTH EDUCATION

Margaret J. Foster

Planning

Question: What are the most common theories reported as being used in the development of physical activity interventions to prevent obesity in adolescents in public schools?
Framework: This question can be framed with the BeHEMoTh (behavior of interest, health context, exclusions, models or theories) framework designed for questions on theories, as shown in box 7.4 (Booth and Carroll, 2015).

TEXTBOX 7.4. FRAMEWORK FOR CASE STUDY 4

Be (behavior of interest): physical activity
H (health context): obese adolescents in public schools
E (exclusions): none
MoTh (models or theories): any

Identifying

Concepts searched: [obesity] and [adolescent] and [physical activity] and [theory]

Bibliographic Databases:

Medline (Ovid)

1. exp obesity/
2. (weight adj2 (gain or loss or change*)).af.
3. (obes* or overweight or over weight).af.
4. ((bmi or body mass index) adj3 (high or gain* or loss* or chang*)).af.
5. or/1–4
6. exp Adolescent/
7. (teen* or adolescen* or youth*).ti,ab.
8. or/6–7
9. exp Motor Activity/ or exp Physical Fitness/ or exp Sports/
10. (physical adj1 (activit* or fitness)).ti,ab.
11. (exercise* or sport* or fitness).ti,ab.
12. (resistance adj1 train*).ti,ab.
13. (weight adj2 lift*).ti,ab.
14. or/9–13
15. exp Psychological Theory/ or exp Social Theory/ or exp Models, Theorectical/
16. (theor* or model*).ti,ab.
17. 15 or 16
18. 5 and 8 and 14 and 17

CINAHL (EBSCO)

((MH "Physical Fitness+") OR (MH "Physical Activity") OR (MH "Sports+") OR (MH "Exercise+") or TI ((physical w1 (activit* or fitness)) or (resistance w1 train*) or (weight w2 lift*) or exercise* or sport* or fitness) or AB ((physical w1 (activit* or fitness)) or (resistance w1 train*) or (weight w2 lift*) or exercise* or sport* or fitness)) AND (((MH "Adolescence") or (MH "Adolescent Health") OR (MH "Adolescent Medicine")) OR TI (teen* or adolescen* or youth*) OR AB (teen* or adolescen* or youth*)) AND (TI (((bmi or body mass index) w3 (high or gain* or loss* or chang*)) OR (obes* or overweight or over weight) OR (weight w2 (gain or loss or change*))) or AB (((bmi or body mass index) w3 (high or gain* or loss* or chang*)) OR (obes* or overweight or over weight) OR (weight w2 (gain or loss or change*)) or (MH "Obesity+"))) AND ((MH "Theory+") OR (MH "Sociological Theory+") OR (MH "Social Learning Theory+") OR (MH "Psychological Theory+") OR (MH "Nursing Theory+") OR (MH "Bandura's Social Cognitive Theory")) OR TI (theory or theories or model or models) OR AB (theory or theories or model or models)

SPORTDiscus (EBSCO)
[(DE "PHYSICAL activity" OR DE "AEROBIC exercises" OR DE "STRENGTH training" OR DE "WEIGHT lifting" OR DE "WEIGHT training" OR DE "BENCH press" OR DE "DEAD lift (Weight lifting)" OR DE "POWERLIFTING" OR DE "SQUAT (Weight lifting)" OR DE "STONE lifting" OR DE "WEIGHT lifting" OR DE "WEIGHT training for boys" OR DE "WEIGHT training for children" OR DE "WEIGHT training for people with disabilities" OR DE "WEIGHT training for women" OR DE "SPORTS" OR DE "AERONAUTICAL sports" OR DE "AMATEUR sports" OR DE "AQUATIC sports" OR DE "BALL games" OR DE "BASEBALL" OR DE "COLLEGE sports" OR DE "CONTACT sports" OR DE "CROSS-training (Sports)" OR DE "DISC golf" OR DE "ENDURANCE sports" OR DE "EXTREME sports" OR DE "GYMNASTICS" OR DE "HOCKEY" OR DE "INDIVIDUAL sports" OR DE "RACKET games" OR DE "RECREATIONAL sports" OR DE "RODEOS" OR DE "ROLLER skating" OR DE "SCHOOL sports" OR DE "SOFTBALL" OR DE "SPORTS competitions" OR DE "SPORTS for children" OR DE "SPORTS for girls" OR DE "SPORTS for youth" OR DE "SPORTS teams" OR DE "TEAM sports" OR DE "WINTER sports") OR TI ((physical w1 (activit* or fitness)) or (resistance w1 train*) or (weight w2 lift*) or exercise* or sport* or fitness) or AB ((physical w1 (activit* or fitness)) or (resistance w1 train*) or (weight w2 lift*) or exercise* or sport* or fitness)] AND [TI (((bmi or body mass index) w3 (high or gain* or loss* or chang*)) OR (obes* or overweight or over weight) OR (weight w2 (gain or loss or change*))) or AB (((bmi or body mass index) w3 (high or gain* or loss* or chang*)) OR (obes* or overweight or over weight) OR (weight w2 (gain or loss or change*))) OR (DE "OBESITY" OR DE "OBESITY in children") OR (DE "OVERWEIGHT teenagers")] AND [DE "TEENAGERS" OR TI (teen* or adolescen* or youth*) OR AB (teen* or adolescen* or youth*)] AND (TI (theory or theories or model or models) OR AB (theory or theories or model or models))

Grey Literature:
Physical Activity Intervention Programs, listed by National Cancer Institute. http://rtips.cancer.gov/rtips/topicPrograms.do?topicId=102268&choice=default

Related Resources

Related reviews to the topic:

Bélanger-Gravel, A., G. Godin, L.-A. Vézina-Im, S. Amireault, and P. Poirier. 2011. "The Effect of Theory-Based Interventions on Physical Activity Participation among Overweight/Obese Individuals: A Systematic Review." *Obesity Reviews: An Official Journal of the International Association for the Study of Obesity* 12 (6): 430–39. doi:10.1111/j.1467-789X.2010.00729.x.

Chilton, R., M. Pearson, and R. Anderson. 2015. "Health Promotion in Schools: A Scoping Review of Systematic Reviews." *Health Education* 115 (3–4): 357–76.

Safron, Magdalena, Aleksandra Cislak, Tania Gaspar, and Aleksandra Luszczynska. 2011. "Effects of School-Based Interventions Targeting Obesity-Related Behaviors and Body Weight Change: A Systematic Umbrella Review." *Behavioral Medicine (Washington, D.C.)* 37 (1): 15–25. doi:10.1080/08964289.2010.543194.

Young, M. D., R. C. Plotnikoff, C. E. Collins, R. Callister, and P. J. Morgan. 2014. "Social Cognitive Theory and Physical Activity: A Systematic Review and Meta-Analysis." *Obesity Reviews: An Official Journal of the International Association for the Study of Obesity* 15 (12): 983–95. doi:10.1111/obr.12225.

Related articles/resources to type of systematic review:

Armstrong, R., E. Waters, N. Jackson, S. Oliver, J. Popay, J. Shepherd, M. Petticrew, et al. 2007. *Guidelines for Systematic Reviews of Health Promotion and Public Health Interventions*. Australia: Melbourne University.

Cavill, N., N. Roberts, and H. Rutter. 2012. *Standard Evaluation Framework for Physical Activity Interventions*. Public Health England Obesity Knowledge and Intelligence Team. https://www.noo.org.uk/core/frameworks/SEF_PA.

Franks, H., N. Hardiker, M. McGrath, and C. McQuarrie. 2012. "Public Health Interventions and Behaviour Change: Reviewing the Grey Literature." *Public Health* 126 (1): 12–17. doi:10.1016/j.puhe.2011.09.023.

CASE STUDY 5: ECONOMIC QUESTIONS WITHIN THE DISCIPLINE OF ENGINEERING

Margaret J. Foster

Planning

Question: What are the most cost-effective methods to mitigate greenhouse gas emissions in truck transportation?
Framework: This question can be framed with the CIMO (context, intervention, mechanisms, outcomes) framework designed for management or policy questions, as shown in box 7.5 (Denyer and Tranfield, 2009).

TEXTBOX 7.5. FRAMEWORK FOR CASE STUDY 5

C (context): truck transportation
I (intervention): mitigation methods for greenhouse gas emissions
M (mechanisms): policies
O (outcomes): economic impacts

Identifying

Concepts searched: [trucks] and [economics] and [greenhouse gases]
Bibliographic Databases:
Compendex

((((({Cost benefit analysis} WN CV) OR ({Cost effectiveness} WN CV) OR ({Cost reduction} WN CV) OR ({Costs} WN CV) OR ({Economics} WN CV))))) or ((($cost AND ($effective OR $analysis OR $reduction)) WN ALL))) and ((((({Chlorofluorocarbons} WN CV) OR ({Freons} WN CV) OR ({Greenhouse gases} WN CV) OR ({Fluorocarbons} WN CV) OR ({Greenhouse effect} WN CV) OR ({Methane} WN CV) OR ({Carbon dioxide} WN CV) OR ({Nitrogen oxides} WN CV) OR ({Ozone} WN CV))))) or ((greenhouse* OR $methane OR {carbon dioxide} OR {nitrous oxide} OR $ozone OR halocarbon* OR $freon OR chlorofluorocarbon*) WN KY)) and (((((({Truck trailers} WN CV) OR ({Truck transportation} WN CV) OR ({Trucks} WN CV) OR ({Tractors (truck)} WN CV) OR ({Trailers—Motor truck*} WN CV))))) or ((((transport* OR trailer*) AND truck*) WN KY)))

Web of Science

[TS=(truck* near/3 (trailer* or transport* or haul* or tractor*))] AND [TS=(cost* or economic*)] AND [TS=(greenhouse or methane or "carbon dioxide" or "nitrous oxide" or ozone* or chlorofluorocarbon* or halocarbon* or freon*)]

Mechanical & Transportation Engineering Abstracts (Proquest)

(SU.EXACT("Trailer-truck combinations") OR SU.EXACT("Truck trailers") OR SU.EXACT("Fleet trucks") OR SU.EXACT("Truck-trailer combinations") OR SU.EXACT("Truck transportation") OR SU.EXACT("Trucks")) OR ab(truck* OR tractor* OR trailer*) AND (SU.EXACT("Greenhouse gases") OR SU.EXACT("Greenhouse effect") OR ab(greenhouse or methane or "carbon dioxide" or "nitrous oxide" or ozone* or chlorofluorocarbon* or halocarbon* or freon*)) AND ((SU.EXACT("Cost benefit analysis")

OR SU.EXACT("Cost analysis") OR SU.EXACT("Minimum cost") OR SU.EXACT("Cost reduction") OR SU.EXACT("Cost effectiveness") OR SU.EXACT("Mitigation costs")) OR ab(cost* or economic*))

TRANSPORT Database (Ovid)

((cost* or economic*) and (greenhouse or methane or "carbon dioxide" or "nitrous oxide" or ozone* or chlorofluorocarbon* or halocarbon* or freon*) and (truck* or tractor* or trailer*)).af.

Grey Literature:

TRID

TRB's Transportation Research Information Services (TRIS) Database and the OECD's Joint Transport Research Centre's International Transport Research Documentation (ITRD) Database:

(truck* AND (cost* or economic*) AND (greenhouse or methane or "carbon dioxide" or "nitrous oxide" or ozone* or chlorofluorocarbon* or halocarbon* or freon*))

National Transportation Library

(kw:truck* OR kw:trailer*) AND (kw:cost OR kw:costs OR kw:economic*) AND (kw:greenhouse OR kw:methane OR kw:"carbon dioxide" OR kw:"nitrous oxide" OR kw:ozone* OR kw:chlorofluorocarbon* OR kw:halocarbon* OR kw:freon*)

New Jersey Environmental Digital Library:

Browse at http://njedl.rutgers.edu

Related Resource

Osif, Bonnie A. 2000. "Transportation Information: A Review of Grey Literature by Format, Language and Availability." *International Journal on Grey Literature* 1 (1): 12–17.

CASE STUDY 6: QUESTION ON RISK OR PROTECTION IN THE PUBLIC HEALTH FIELD

Sarah T. Jewell

Planning

Question: What are the risk factors that increase adolescent females' chance of developing human papillomaviruses (HPV)?

Framework: This question can be framed with the PEO (population, exposure, outcome), as shown in box 7.6 (Kahn et al. 2003).

TEXTBOX 7.6. FRAMEWORK FOR CASE STUDY 6

P (population): adolescent females
E (exposure): risk factors
O (outcome): diagnosis of a human papillomavirus

Identifying

Concepts searched: [adolescent] and [human papillomaviruses] and [risk]
Bibliographic Databases:
PubMed
(((("Risk"[Mesh] OR "Risk Factors"[Mesh]) OR risk*[Title/Abstract])) AND (("Papillomaviridae"[Mesh]) OR (hpv[Title/Abstract] OR Papillomaviruses[Title/Abstract]))) AND (("Adolescent"[Mesh]) OR (adolescen*[Title/Abstract] OR teen*[Title/Abstract] OR youth*[Title/Abstract]))
CINAHL (EBSCO)
[(MH "Adolescence+") OR TI (adolescen* or teen* or youth*) OR AB (adolescen* or teen* or youth*)] AND [(MH "Risk Factors+") OR TI risk* OR AB risk*] AND [(MH "Papillomaviruses") OR TI (hpv or Papillomaviruses) OR AB (hpv or Papillomaviruses)]
Embase (Ovid)
[exp papillomaviridae/ or (Papillomaviruses or hpv).ti,ab.] AND [exp adolescent/ or
(adolescen* or teen* or youth*).ti,ab.] AND [exp risk/ or (risk*).ti,ab.]
Grey Literature:
- National Foundation for Infectious Diseases: http://http://www.nfid.org/publications
- Clinicaltrials.gov

Hand Searching:
- *Virus Research*
- *Vaccine*

Related Resources

Armijo-Olivo, Susan, Carla R. Stiles, Neil A. Hagen, Patricia D. Biondo, and Greta G. Cummings. 2012. "Assessment of Study Quality for Systematic Reviews: A Comparison of the Cochrane Collaboration Risk of Bias Tool and the Effective Public Health Practice Project Quality Assessment Tool: Methodological Re-

search." *Journal of Evaluation in Clinical Practice* 18 (1): 12–18. doi:10.1111/j.1365-2753.2010.01516.x.
Jackson, N., and E. Waters. 2005. "Criteria for the Systematic Review of Health Promotion and Public Health Interventions." *Health Promotion International* 20 (4): 367–74. doi:10.1093/heapro/dai022.

CASE STUDY 7: POLICY QUESTION IN THE FIELD OF AGRICULTURE

Jenni Simmonsen

Planning

Question: What are the environmental impacts of trap-neuter-return methods aimed at managing free-roaming cat populations?
Framework: This question can be framed with the SPICE (setting perspective/population, intervention, comparison, evaluation) framework, as detailed in box 7.7 (Booth 2006).

TEXTBOX 7.7. FRAMEWORK FOR CASE STUDY 7

S (setting): citics
P (perspective/population): animal control offices
I (intervention): city policy to alter and return cats to roam free
C (comparison): no policy
E (evaluation): decreased population of cats

Identification

Concepts in search: [environmental impacts] and [population control] and [domesticated cats]
Bibliographic Databases:
CAB Abstracts (Ovid)
(cat.af OR cats.af OR feline.af OR Felis.bt) AND ("population control."af OR "population management."af OR "trap-neuter-return."af OR TNR.af OR trap.af OR contracep*.af OR "birth control."af OR steril*.af OR "fertility control."af OR neuter.af OR spay.af) AND (*predation OR "species diversity" OR environ* OR "wildlife management."sh OR "wildlife

conservation."sh OR "species decline."af OR "ecol* consequenc*."af OR "ecol* impact."af)

AGRICOLA (EBSCO)

TX (cat OR cats OR Felis OR feline) AND TX ("population control" OR "population management" OR "trap-neuter-return" OR TNR OR trap OR contracep* OR "birth control" OR steril* OR "fertility control" OR neuter OR spay) AND TX (*predation OR "species diversity" OR environ* OR "wildlife management" OR "wildlife conservation" OR "species decline" OR "ecol* consequenc*" OR "ecol* impact")

PubMed

(((("Felidae"[Mesh] OR cat OR cats OR Felis OR feline))) AND (("Contraception"[Mesh] OR "Population Control"[Mesh] OR "population management" OR "trap-neuter-return" OR TNR OR trap OR "birth control" OR sterili* OR "fertility control" OR neuter OR spay))) AND (("Predatory Behavior"[Mesh] OR "Environment"[Mesh] OR *predation OR "species diversity" OR environ* OR "wildlife management" OR "wildlife conservation" OR "species decline" OR ecol* OR "population dynamics"))

Wildlife & Ecology Studies Worldwide (EBSCO)

TX (cat OR cats OR Felis OR feline) AND TX ("population control" OR "population management" OR "trap-neuter-return" OR TNR OR trap OR contracep* OR "birth control" OR steril* OR "fertility control" OR neuter OR spay) AND TX (*predation OR "species diversity" OR environ* OR "wildlife management" OR "wildlife conservation" OR "species decline" OR "ecol* consequenc*" OR "ecol* impact")

Environmental Sciences & Pollution Management (ProQuest)

(all(cat) OR all(cats) OR all(Felis) OR all(feline)) AND (all("population control") OR all("population management") OR all("trap-neuter-return") OR all(TNR) OR all(trap) OR all(contracep*) OR all("birth control") OR all(steril*) OR all("fertility control") OR all(neuter) OR all(spay)) AND (all(#predation) OR all(predat*) OR all("species diversity") OR all(environ*) OR all("wildlife management") OR all("wildlife conservation") OR all("species decline") OR all("ecol* consequenc*") OR all("ecol* impact"))

In addition, search:

- ProQuest Dissertations & Theses Global
- Scopus

Grey Literature:

- Where discoverable, county/city animal shelter or wildlife management reports may provide additional studies.

- Grey literature databases (e.g., OpenGrey: http://www.opengrey.eu) might also assist in locating studies.
- Citations could also be requested through known researchers and state or national veterinary, animal control, and wildlife management listservs.

Related Resources

Standards, guides, or organizations related to the topic/discipline area:

Campbell or Cochrane Collaboration reporting standards are commonly used for systematic reviews in agriculture. Relatively few guides are available to assist specifically with systematic reviews in agriculture disciplines. Examples include the following:

- The Collaboration for Environmental Evidence (http://www.environmen talevidence.org) provides guidelines for conducting systematic reviews in environmental management.
- 2010. "The European Food Safety Authority has Published Guidance for Food and Feed Safety Systematic Reviews: European Food Safety Authority." *EFSA Journal*, 8 (6): 1637. doi:10.2903/j.efsa.2010.1637.
- Sargeant, J. M., M. Amezcua, A. Rajic, and L. Waddell. 2005. *A Guide to Conducting Systematic Reviews in Agri-Food Public Health.*
- Young, Ian, Ashley Kerr, Lisa Waddell, Mai T. Pham, Judy Greig, Scott A. McEwen, and Andrijana Rajić. 2014. "A Guide for Developing Plain-Language and Contextual Summaries of Systematic Reviews in Agri-Food Public Health." *Foodborne Pathogens and Disease* 11 (12): 930–937. doi:10.1089/fpd.2014.1807.

Several organizations outside traditional academic agricultural librarianship leverage existing protocols, standards, and guides to provide systematic review services, develop systematic reviews, or foster evidence-based practice:

- The Centre for Evidence Based Agriculture at Harper Adams University provides agri-food-related systematic review services (http://www.harper -adams.ac.uk/initiatives/centre-evidence-based-agriculture)
- The Centre for Agriculture and Biosciences International (CABI) is working to conduct systematic reviews related to agriculture (http://www.cabi .org/services/knowledge-management-services/systematic-reviews)
- The Center for International Forestry Research has an Evidence-Based Forestry Initiative to promote systematic reviews in this discipline (http:// www1.cifor.org/ebf/home.html)

References important to agriculture systematic reviews:
For some practical notes to consider when evaluating evidence to be used in agriculture-related systematic reviews, consider the following:

- Virgona, Jim, and Geoff Daniel. 2011. "Evidence-Based Agriculture—Can We Get There?" *Agricultural Science* 23 (1): 19–25.
- In 2014, the journal *Zoonoses & Public Health* devoted a special issue to animal-related systematic reviews as listed in case study 1.
- The Collaboration for Environmental Evidence developed and manages an Environmental Evidence Library and publishes the open access journal *Environmental Evidence*: http://www.environmentalevidence.org.

CASE STUDY 8: ADVERSE EFFECTS IN THE PHARMACEUTICAL FIELD

Sarah T. Jewell

Planning

Question: What are the long-term adverse effects of Celebrex in elderly patients?
Framework: This question can be framed with the PICOT format as detailed in box 7.8 (Richardson et al. 1995).

TEXTBOX 7.8. FRAMEWORK FOR CASE STUDY 8

P (population): patients over sixty
I (intervention): Celebrex
C (comparison): does not apply
O (outcome): adverse effects
T (time): after at least one year of usage

Identifying

Concepts searched: [elderly] and [celebrex] and [adverse effects]

Bibliographic Databases:

EMBASE (Ovid)

1. celecoxib/
2. (celecoxib or artroxil or caditar or celcox or celebra or celebrex or celecox or celib or coxel or coxid or dilox or eliflam or lexfin or onsenal or sc58635 or ym177 or zycel).mp.
3. 1 or 2
4. (ae or si or to or co).fs.
5. (safe or safety).ti,ab.
6. side effect$.ti,ab.
7. ((adverse or undesirable or harm$ or serious or toxic) adj3 (effect$ or reaction$ or event$ or outcome$)).ti,ab.
8. exp adverse drug reaction/ or exp drug toxicity/ or exp intoxication/ or exp drug safety/ or exp drug monitoring/ or exp drug hypersensitivity/ or exp postmarketing surveillance/ or exp drug surveillance program/ or exp phase iv clinical trial/
9. (toxicity or complication$ or noxious or tolerability).ti,ab.
10. exp postoperative complication/ or exp Peroperative Complication/ or exp Perioperative Complication/
11. or/4–10
12. aged/
13. (elderly or aged).mp.
13. 12 or 13
14. 3 and 11 and 13

MEDLINE (Ovid)

1. Celecoxib/
2. (celecoxib or artroxil or caditar or celcox or celebra or celebrex or celecox or celib or coxel or coxid or dilox or eliflam or lexfin or onsenal or sc58635 or ym177 or zycel).mp.
3. 1 or 2
4. (ae or to or po or co).fs.
5. (safe or safety).ti,ab.
6. side effect$.ti,ab.
7. ((adverse or undesirable or harms$ or serious or toxic) adj3 (effect$ or reaction$ or event$ or outcome$)).ti,ab.
8. exp product surveillance, postmarketing/ or exp adverse drug reaction reporting systems/ or exp clinical trials, phase iv/ or exp poisoning/ or exp substance-related disorders/ or exp drug toxicity/ or exp abnormalities, drug induced/ or exp drug monitoring/ or exp drug hypersensitivity/
9. (toxicity or complication$ or noxious or tolerability).ti,ab.
10. exp Postoperative Complications/ or exp Intraoperative Complications/

11. or/ 4–10
12. Aged/
13. (elderly or aged).mp.
14. 12 or 13
15. 3 and 11 and 14

Grey Literature:

- ClinicalTrials.gov
- FDA Medwatch: http://www.fda.gov/medwatch/index.html
- Database of Adverse Event Notifications (DAEN) from Australian government Department of Health: https://www.tga.gov.au/database-adverse-event-notifications-daen
- Derwent Drug File

Hand Searching:

- *BMC Clinical Pharmacology, Drug Safety*
- *Pharmacoepidemiology & Drug Safety*

Related Resources

The search filter for adverse effects for the Embase and Medline searches above was copied from the *British Medical Journal* list of search filters, found at http://clinicalevidence.bmj.com/x/set/static/ebm/learn/665076.html.

Golder, Su, and Yoon Loke. 2009. "Search Strategies to Identify Information on Adverse Effects: A Systematic Review." *JMLA: Journal of the Medical Library Association* 97 (2): 84–92. doi:10.3163/1536-5050.97.2.004.

Golder, Su, and Yoon K. Loke. 2010. "Sources of Information on Adverse Effects: A Systematic Review." *Health Information and Libraries Journal* 27 (3): 176–90. doi:10.1111/j.1471-1842.2010.00901.x.

Golder, Su, Yoon Loke, and Heather M. McIntosh. 2008. "Poor Reporting and Inadequate Searches Were Apparent in Systematic Reviews of Adverse Effects." *Journal of Clinical Epidemiology* 61 (5): 440–48. doi:10.1016/j.jclinepi.2007.06.005.

———. 2006. "Room for Improvement? A Survey of the Methods used in Systematic Reviews of Adverse Effects." *BMC Medical Research Methodology* 6:3. doi:10.1186/1471-2288-6-3.

Golder, Su, Yoon K. Loke, Kath Wright, and Carmelo Sterrantino. 2016. "Most Systematic Reviews of Adverse Effects Did Not Include Unpublished Data." *Journal of Clinical Epidemiology*. doi:10.1016/j.jclinepi.2016.05.003.

Loke, Yoon K., Deirdre Price, Andrew Herxheimer, and Cochrane Adverse Effects Methods Group. 2007. "Systematic Reviews of Adverse Effects: Framework for a Structured Approach." *BMC Medical Research Methodology* 7:32. doi:10.1186/1471-2288-7-32.

Zorzela, Liliane, Su Golder, Yali Liu, Karen Pilkington, Lisa Hartling, Ari Joffe, Yoon Loke, and Sunita Vohra. 2014. "Quality of Reporting in Systematic Reviews of Adverse Events: Systematic Review." *BMJ (Clinical Research Ed.)* 348:f7668.

CASE STUDY 9: DIAGNOSIS QUESTION IN THE EDUCATION FIELD

Sarah T. Jewell

Planning

Question: What is the best screening tool for diagnosing dyslexia children in K–12 educational settings?
Framework: This question can be framed with the PICO format, adapted for diagnostic questions, as detailed in box 7.9 (Kim, Lee, Choi, Huh, and Park, 2015).

TEXTBOX 7.9. FRAMEWORK FOR CASE STUDY 9

P (population): elementary school children suspected of dyslexia
I (index tests): educational diagnosis
C (comparator tests): clinical diagnosis
O (outcome): correct diagnosis

Identifying

Concepts searched: [dyslexia] and [diagnosis]
Bibliographic Databases:
ERIC (EBSCO)
(DE "Dyslexia" OR TI (dyslexi*) OR AB(dylexi*)) AND (DE "Educational Diagnosis OR TI (diagnos*) OR AB(diagnos*))
PsycINFO (EBSCO)
(DE "Dyslexia" OR TI (dyslexi*) OR AB(dylexi*)) AND (DE "Diagnosis" OR DE "Educational Diagnosis" TI (diagnos*) OR AB(diagnos*))
Conference Abstracts:
- International Dyslexia Association
- Dyslexia Foundation
- European Dyslexia Association

Hand Searching:
- *Learning Disabilities Research and Practice*
- *Dyslexia*
- *Annals of Dyslexia*

Related Resources

Andrews, Richard. 2005. "The Place of Systematic Reviews in Education Research." *British Journal of Educational Studies* 53 (4): 399–416.
Andrews, Richard, and Wynne Harlen. 2006. "Issues in Synthesizing Research in Education." *Educational Research* 48 (3): 287–99.
Bearman, Margaret, Calvin D. Smith, Angela Carbone, Susan Slade, Chi Baik, Marnie Hughes-Warrington, and David L. Neumann. 2012. "Systematic Review Methodology in Higher Education." *Higher Education Research and Development* 31 (5): 625–40.
Bennett, Judith, Fred Lubben, Sylvia Hogarth, and Bob Campbell. 2005. "Systematic Reviews of Research in Science Education: Rigour or Rigidity?" *International Journal of Science Education* 27 (4): 387–406.
Campbell, J. M., M. Klugar, S. Ding, D. P. Carmody, S. J. Hakonsen, Y. T. Jardotte, S. White, and Z. Munn. 2015. *The Systematic Review of Studies of Diagnostic Test Accuracy*. Adelaide, Australia: Joanna Briggs Institute.
Hempenstall, Kerry. 2014. "What Works? Evidence-Based Practice in Education Is Complex." *Australian Journal of Learning Difficulties* 19 (2): 113–27.
Institute of Education Sciences. 2014. *WWC Procedures and Standards Handbook*: U.S. Department of Education.
Social Science Research Unit, Institute of Education. 2010. *EPPI-Centre Methods for Conducting Systematic Reviews*. London: University of London.

CONCLUSION

Working examples is one way to build skills in developing searches for systematic reviews. The process is greatly enhanced by getting feedback from others. In addition, as disciplines and topics can vary widely, it is important to ask for input from librarians with expertise in that subject as well. This provides context and information that would otherwise be missed.

REFERENCES

Booth, Andrew. 2006. "Clear and Present Questions: Formulating Questions for Evidence Based Practice." *Library Hi Tech* 24 (3): 355–68.
Booth, Andrew, and Christopher Carroll. 2015. "Systematic Searching for Theory to Inform Systematic Reviews: Is It Feasible? Is It Desirable?" *Health Information and Libraries Journal* 32 (3): 220–35.
Cooke, A., D. Smith, and A. Booth. 2012. "Beyond PICO: The SPIDER Tool for Qualitative Evidence Synthesis." *Qualitative Health Research* 22 (10): 1435–43. doi:10.1177/1049732312452938.

Denyer, David, and David Tranfield. "Producing a Systematic Review." In the *Sage Handbook of Organizational Research Methods*, ed. D. Buchanan and A. Bryman, 671–89. Los Angeles: Sage Publications, 2009.

Kahn, K. S., R. Kunz, J. Kleijnen, and G. Antes. 2003. *Systematic Reviews to Support Evidence-Based Medicine: How to Review and Apply Findings of Health Care Research*. London: RSM Press.

Kim, Kyung Won, Juneyoung Lee, Sang Hyun Choi, Jimi Huh, and Seong Ho Park. 2015. "Systematic Review and Meta-Analysis of Studies Evaluating Diagnostic Test Accuracy: A Practical Review for Clinical Researchers—Part I. General Guidance and Tips." *Korean Journal of Radiology* 16 (6): 1175–87.

Richardson, W. S., M. C. Wilson, J. Nishikawa, and R. S. Hayward. 1995. "The Well-Built Clinical Question: A Key to Evidence-Based Decisions." *ACP Journal Club* 123 (3): 12.

Chapter Eight

Evaluating

Study Selection and Critical Appraisal

Misa Mi

If there was one life skill everyone on the planet needed, it was the ability to think with critical objectivity.

—Josh Lanyon

OBJECTIVES

- Explain the process of screening search results for a systematic review using predefined selection/eligibility criteria
- Discuss ways of making the study selection process systematic and transparent
- Recognize strategies for handling issues in the selection process
- Discuss the process of critical appraisal of included studies for the review
- Select and apply appropriate quality assessment tools for critical appraisal of included studies
- Identify librarians' roles in the selection and critical appraisal process

OVERVIEW

As articles are retrieved, the evaluation process begins with a series of processes: screening by title/abstract, selection by reading the full text of study reports, and finally evaluating the methods and reporting of potential studies. As Josh Lanyon said, the ability for critical thinking is a vital skill in the process. In addition, a solid grasp of research design and potential threats to validity is also required. Validity is "the degree to which we can accept the evidence as trustworthy and believable" (Pearson, Field, and Jordan 2009). Each of the processes has standards and best practices that should be considered when planning, conducting, and reporting this step. Critical appraisal is the most important and needs the most time in planning and selecting appropriate methods—such as validated risk of bias checklists.

SELECTING STUDIES FOR INCLUSION

Following the step of literature searches, reviewers start the next step of the systematic review process—selecting studies and making decisions about which studies to include or exclude in a review according to prespecified inclusion/exclusion (selection/eligibility) criteria. The decisions are very influential in the review process. What follows offers a step-by-step process for selecting studies for inclusion (see box 8.1) and introduces a few approaches to handling issues encountered in the selection process. The potential opportunities for librarians during this process are described in librarian's corner 8.1.

LIBRARIAN'S CORNER 8.1. LIBRARIAN ROLES IN SCREENING AND SELECTING STUDIES

- Assist client in identifying and choosing the best tool for screening abstracts
- Ensure quality control over process by checking that all citations are screened and sorted appropriately, pointing out disagreements
- Screen articles as a member of the review team (as appropriate)
- Serve as project manager, dividing up the articles between review team members

Screening by Title and Abstract

Comprehensive literature searches may yield a potentially large evidence base in a review topic area. When there is a large retrieval with several thousand search results or citations, the selection process may seem very daunting. To start the process, the first step is to sift titles from searches, remove clearly irrelevant and duplicate studies, and leave a subset of studies to be screened by two reviewers in the subsequent screening phases. During the initial screening phase, a librarian can be invited to examine a sample of the excluded studies to check that the process is working and that no relevant citations are inadvertently removed. By doing that, reviewers can assure that important studies are not missed and the eligibility criteria are appropriately applied (Petticrew and Roberts 2006). The key to this process is that authors are looking for reasons to exclude a citation, not to keep it, as abstracts provide a limited amount of information about the study.

TEXTBOX 8.1. PROCESS OF STUDY SELECTION

Step 1: De-duplicate citations and pilot test eligibility criteria
Step 2: Screen titles and abstracts identified via searches using eligibility criteria
Step 3: Obtain full-text articles of all potentially relevant studies
Step 4: Select full-text articles for inclusion in a review using eligibility criteria
Step 5: Report results of the selection process based on the PRISMA statement
Adapted from Liberati et al. 2009. "The PRISMA Statement for Reporting Systematic Reviews and Meta-Analyses of Studies That Evaluate Health Care Interventions: Explanation and Elaboration." *PLoS Med* 6 (7): e1000100.

Following the initial title screening to remove irrelevant and duplicate studies, reviewers examine abstracts of any studies when there is any doubt on the relevance of the studies or it is impossible to judge relevance from their titles alone (Booth, Papaioannou, and Sutton 2012). Citations with abstracts that seem potentially relevant to the selection criteria should be provisionally included as candidates for full-text screening. Citations that are apparently irrelevant should be excluded from the lists at this phase, and the number of citations excluded should be documented. As the inclusion/exclusion decisions involve judgments that may vary from one reviewer to another, it is desirable for more than one reviewer to participate in the abstract screening process. The involvement of two or more reviewers may help ensure reproducible assessments made in the process and reduce the possibility that potentially relevant studies will be removed (Morton et al. 2011).

Once the reviewers have identified potentially relevant studies, they locate and obtain full-text articles, organize, and store them for further screening. It has been revealed that reports with statistically significant results are more likely to get published than those with nonsignificant findings (Smith

1980). To minimize outcome reporting or publication bias in a review, it is advisable that the selection process include both published and unpublished reports (Cooper 2010). If abstracts from certain conferences or proceedings that clearly meet the selection criteria are included for the full-text screening, reviewers may need to correspond with the principal investigators of these abstracts to obtain unpublished manuscripts, data on outcomes of interest, or other relevant information (e.g., research methods). Raw data that appear as a secondary interest to the investigators of a primary study but are relevant to the selection criteria may be acquired during the process.

Screening Full-Text Articles

The output of citations from the screening process may vary from one reviewer to another (Khan et al. 2011). Given that citations contain limited information on the content of potentially relevant articles, uncertainties on studies may remain following abstract screening. Thus, full-text articles of all citations considered potentially relevant by each reviewer should be obtained for full-text screening. Information contained in each article should be assessed against the selection criteria; articles that do not meet any of the selection criteria should be excluded.

Existing systematic review guides emphasize the importance of more than one reviewer screening articles in entirety independently and in duplicate to minimize biases and reduce the risk of errors of human judgment in the selection process (Haase 2011; Morton et al. 2011). Furthermore, the screening process needs to be systematic and transparent because inclusion decisions made at this full-text screening phase are influential in the review. It is recommended that the selection criteria be pilot tested on a sample set of full-text articles (e.g., ten to twelve articles) (Higgins and Green 2008). The pilot test can determine if reviewers apply the selection criteria in a consistent fashion in the independent and duplicate screening process. It is also a good practice for reviewers to keep note of the number of studies on which they agree and disagree. If the agreement between the two reviewers is poor in the pilot test, the prespecified selection criteria may need to be clarified and revised.

It is important that at the full-text screening stage, at least one reviewer is knowledgeable of the subject or the topic under review. However, content experts in a discipline or research field may possess preconceived ideas or opinions or they may have established collaborative relationships with other researchers. As a result, content experts may be susceptible to possible biases that likely affect their judgment of the value and relevance of individual studies or their selection of studies with opposing views. Having another reviewer who is not a content expert may offer an advantage to the selection process (Higgins and Green 2008).

Measuring Selection Agreement

Given that the inclusion/exclusion decisions made by each reviewer may be subjective and are likely susceptible to individual selection biases, disagreements may arise concerning the study selection among the reviewers at the full-text screening stage. Reviewers should compare notes and resolve disagreements by consensus. In any event, when reviewers fail to reach a consensus due to a difference in interpretation, the disagreement may require arbitration by a third reader/reviewer who serves as a tiebreaker between two reviewers. There are formal measures used to determine the rate of agreement in inclusion/exclusion decisions by multiple reviewers (e.g., the kappa statistic). The kappa statistic, albeit it is not required for all systematic reviews, may be calculated to measure the level of agreement between two reviewers, with the most useful kappa being Gwet's AC1. The application of kappa statistics and interpretation of values can be found in other works (Wongpakaran et al. 2013).

Identifying and Selecting Studies from Duplicate Publications

When screening citations, reviewers may encounter multiple publications of the same study. These publications may be duplicates that can introduce substantial biases to the conclusions of data synthesis if they are inadvertently included in the selection process. Studies (e.g., clinical trials of drugs) reporting positive or greater treatment effects are more likely to be duplicated. Data from these duplicates that are analyzed more than once in meta-analysis can lead to overestimation of treatment efficacy (Tramer et al. 1997).

To detect possible duplicate publications, reviewers need to compare studies by examining author names, the location and setting of a given study, a detailed description of the intervention, sample sizes, baseline data, and date and duration of the study. If there is uncertainty about duplication, it may be necessary to contact the authors of reports for clarification. When it comes to making inclusion/exclusion decisions, one approach is to link together multiple reports of the same study; another is to examine information available in multiple reports to determine which studies are eligible for inclusion (Higgins and Green 2008). Khan et al. suggest that only the data from the largest, most complete report with the longest follow-up be counted once (Khan et al. 2011).

Documentation

The number of articles excluded at each phase of the selection process should be documented. The reason for exclusion at the full-text screening stage should be recorded and detailed for the sake of maintaining a transparent procedure and for the purpose of subsequent reporting of the screening procedure. The documentation also allows for justification for the selection decisions made at the full-text screening stage and offers answers to any possible queries regarding particular articles excluded from the review (Booth, Papaioannou, and Sutton 2012). A brief list of excluded full-text articles along with primary reasons for exclusion may be included as an appendix when submitting a report of a systematic review for publication. Requirements for the list and reasons for exclusion may vary from one journal to another. However, a diagram or flowchart illustrating the selection decision-making process is needed in a final report of data synthesis to show the number of duplicate articles removed, articles excluded at each screening phase, and the primary reason for each full-text article excluded for the review. Figure 8.1 shows an example of an abbreviated flowchart of the study selection process adapted from the PRISMA statement for reporting systematic reviews.

The conduct of a successful review requires a mechanism for effective project management and documentation of the selection process. Librarians are well positioned to take charge of the process in relation to information management and process documentation. A few examples of tasks they undertake include importing citations to a reference management software program (e.g., EndNote) and exporting lists of citations from EndNote into an Excel spreadsheet, where reviewers can easily write notes on procure-

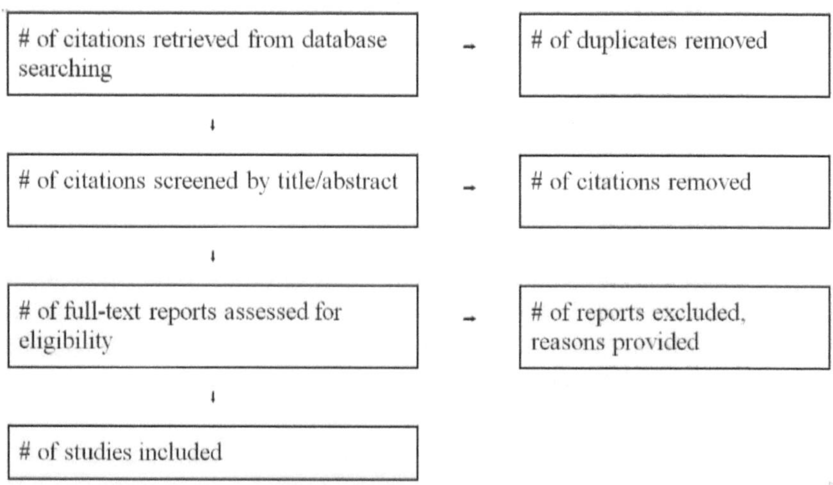

Figure 8.1. Example of PRISMA flowchart
Adapted from Alessandro et al. 2009. "The PRISMA statement for reporting systematic reviews and meta-analyses of studies that evaluate health care interventions: explanation and elaboration." *PLoS Med* 6 (7): e1000100. doi: 10.1371/journal.pmed.1000100.

ment status (whether full-text articles have been requested and obtained) as well as information on screening and eligibility decisions, including specific reasons for exclusion of each citation. Librarians can also directly tag the citations with keywords at the abstract and full-text screening phases or attach available full-text articles in PDF to individual references in EndNote. The practice makes it quick and easy to retrieve a list of included studies and provides an audit trail of inclusion/exclusion decisions for quality control of the procedure (Booth, Papaioannou, and Sutton 2012).

CRITICAL APPRAISAL

Following the selection process is critical appraisal that involves a risk of bias assessment or quality assessment of the final set of included full-text articles. This is an essential step in conducting a systematic review. Quality refers to the degree to which a study employs measures to reduce bias and error in its design, conduct, and analysis (Khan et al. 2011). "The purpose of study quality assessment is to capture and analyze variations among the included studies in terms of their credibility and vulnerability to various sources of bias" (Littell, Corcoran, and Pillai 2008). Critical appraisal is a process of systematically evaluating the validity of research and its relevance to a specific review question (Nelson 2014).

There are certain measures that reviewers can take to ensure a transparent and systematic process: (1) creating a review protocol that provides a clear description of how to assess quality, (2) selecting a validated critical appraisal tool, (3) testing the tool with a sample of selected articles, and (4) involving two or more reviewers in the appraisal process for the sake of quality control of the critical appraisal process. Box 8.2 summarizes general steps in conducting critical appraisal of included studies for a review.

TEXTBOX 8.2. KEY STEPS INVOLVED IN CRITICAL APPRAISAL

Step 1: Note the type of study design in included studies based on a review question
Step 2: Identify a valid quality assessment tool appropriate for a review
Step 3: Two or more reviewers test the tool with a sample of included studies
Step 4: Reviewers carry out critical appraisal of included studies independently and in duplicate
Step 5: Tabulate and summarize results of critical appraisal

Tools for Critical Appraisal

In the process of critical appraisal, it is important to ensure the reliability of an assessment instrument (e.g., checklist) for assessing the quality of included studies to avoid subjectivity and errors when extracting information about quality from each study. A great number and variety of assessment tools in the form of scales or checklists have been proposed and published for use in systematic reviews. Many tools are scales that reviewers use to score various components of a study's design, conduct, and analysis. Assessment tools can also be checklists that contain a list of specific questions with fixed response options which prompt reviewers to make an evaluative judgment on the validity of a study (Gough, Oliver, and Thomas 2012). Reviewers should bear in mind that a widely used assessment tool doesn't mean the tool will produce the "right" answer about the validity of a study addressing a specific research question.

Herbison and colleagues reviewed forty-three quality scales used to score the quality of randomized controlled trials. They found that none of the scales appeared to be valid measures of the quality of the trials. Most of the scales reviewed had no justification for what they included in the scales, and many included scale items that may not address any bias in studies (Herbison, Hay-Smith, and Gillespie 2006). Other researchers found that among twenty-five scales and nine checklists reviewed, many instruments contained items that were not directly related to internal validity (Moher et al. 1995; Moher, Jadad, and Tugwell 1996). Different scales have been shown to provide unreliable assessments of internal validity because these scales may lead to very different evaluation results when scoring the quality of the same studies. Jüni et al. warned that the single-score approach or the use of summary scores to identify randomized trials of high quality is problematic (Jüni et al. 1999). Herbison, Hay-Smith, and Gillespie (2006) state that "it is a mistake to assign meaning to the result of a quality score." The practice of using overall quality scales in meta-analysis should be discarded (Littell, Corcoran, and Pillai 2008). It is recommended that study qualities should be assessed individually rather than being summarized into total quality scores using assessment scales (Higgins and Green 2008; Shadish and Myers 2004). When it comes to judging the quality of individual studies, the assessment should focus on individual study features such as specific study design and implementation issues that are prone to risks of bias in studies.

Once the risk of bias has been assessed, then the reviewers "must confront the contentious issue whether studies of inferior quality are to be included" (Marchevsky and Wick 2011). Some methodologists suggest that synthesizing studies of high quality with those of low quality can lead to incorrect conclusions (Garg, Hackam, and Tonelli, 2008). Others contend that including all relevant studies despite quality issues allows for more studies varied by sample, setting, and other situations (Marchevsky and Wick 2011). In addition, since quality scales are based on the report of a study and not necessarily actually representative of how well an experiment was carried out, there is some criticism of this measure. For example, more recent studies may be more likely to be assessed as of higher quality, since reporting standards have evolved and now dictate that researchers detail their methods more explicitly. If studies with high risk of bias are included, the variations in quality need to be considered during the synthesis and analysis. Some experts have suggested including minimum quality standard as part of the eligibility criteria. This issue continues to be debated in the synthesis methodology literature.

In determining a critical appraisal tool for quality assessment, reviewers need to consider generic study design–based items or features and develop assessment tools customized for different study designs relevant to the type of review question or the outcomes measured in studies. For a review addressing a question on an intervention, only randomized control trials may be selected (Glasziou 2001). However, blinding may not be possible for studies investigating certain surgical procedures, and hence assessment criteria may be confined to the study design features such as randomization and adequate follow-up. It should be noted that blinding is highly crucial in studies with subjective outcomes, but not so much in those with objective outcomes (Khan et al. 2011).

Following are a few approaches to critical appraisal of studies of methodological designs commonly used in research reports across various disciplines.

Assessing Randomized Studies

Randomized studies are experimental research that involves the manipulation of at least one test treatment or intervention (independent variable) followed by observing the effects of the manipulation on one or more dependent variables (Gall, Borg, and Gall 2007). This type of research design is also called a pretest-posttest control group design or posttest-only control group design in educational research or other fields of research. The intervention can be a therapy, procedure, service, or educational program. The quality of a systematic review depends on the validity of included randomized studies. Evaluation of the validity of studies has an indelible influence on the analysis, interpretation, and conclusions of a systematic review because a meta-analysis of invalid or biased studies may produce spurious results or lead to underestimation or overestimation of the true intervention effect (a false positive or negative conclusion).

It is clear that an inverse relationship exists between bias and quality: studies with greater risks of bias are generally of lower quality; their results are more likely to be misleading (Nelson 2014) or to overestimate intervention effects (Khan, Daya, and Jadad 1996; Petticrew and Roberts 2006). It is necessary for reviewers to understand key biases so that they can recognize

Table 8.1. Common risks of bias in randomized studies

Type of bias	*Description*	*Domain/quality assessment item*
Selection bias	Bias due to the assignment of study participants to groups in a way resulting in systematic differences in important baseline characteristics, prognosis, or responsiveness to treatment	• Generation of random sequence for allocating participants to groups • Allocation concealed in advance of or during enrollment • Assessing baseline differences to evaluate success of randomization and need to perform statistical adjustment • Use of intention-to-treat analysis
Performance bias	Bias resulted from differential provision of care or instruction provided, follow-up, or exposure to factors, rather than the intervention being investigated	• Blinding of study participants, care providers, research personnel
Attrition bias	Bias due to loss to follow-up, when participants lost to follow-up differ systematically from those who remain in the study	• Reporting of loss to follow-up • Magnitude of loss to follow-up, including differences across groups • Intention-to-treat analysis (any description of withdrawals or dropouts for such an analysis) • Use of statistical methods to account for missing data
Measurement bias	Bias related to differential assessment of outcomes due to knowledge of the intervention received	• Blinding of outcomes assessors, data analysts, and research personnel as appropriate to the study
Reporting bias	Bias due to a tendency to underreport results, based on the direction or statistical significance of those results	• Report all prespecified primary and important secondary outcomes and analyses, regardless of direction of effect or statistical significance

Source: Higgins and Green 2008; Khan et al. 2011; Nelson 2014

any of them during their critical appraisal of included studies. A few common or generic biases that impact the internal validity of an intervention study include selection bias, performance bias, measurement bias, attrition bias, and reporting bias (Boland, Cherry, and Dickson 2014). Table 8.1 lists five common biases with brief descriptions and associated relevant domains or assessment items for making judgments about risk of bias in randomized studies (Higgins and Green 2008; Nelson 2014).

Given that assessment criteria for randomized studies are straightforward and have been fully developed and validated, answering the specific questions listed in box 8.3 may fulfill the minimum assessment requirement of critical appraisal. In making judgments using the checklist in box 8.3, reviewers can answer each specific question on the basis of descriptions provided in study reports as "Adequate" or "Yes" for a low risk of bias, "No" for high risk of bias, or "Unclear" for insufficient data or no information provided. Other sources of bias (see chapter 9 for more details) will need to be considered in critical appraisal, depending on types of included studies and review questions.

TEXTBOX 8.3. CHECKLIST FOR APPRAISING RANDOMIZED STUDIES

Assessment questions/items	*Yes*	*No*	*Unclear*	*N/A*
1. Was the assignment of participants to treatment truly randomized?	☐	☐	☐	☐
2. Was randomization concealed?	☐	☐	☐	☐
3. Were participants and research personnel blind to the treatment?	☐	☐	☐	☐
4. Were the outcomes of participants who withdrew described and included in the analysis?	☐	☐	☐	☐
5. Were those assessing outcomes blind to the treatment allocation?	☐	☐	☐	☐
6. Were participants in study groups comparable at baseline or at the start of the study?	☐	☐	☐	☐
7. Was appropriate statistical analysis used?	☐	☐	☐	☐
8. Were outcomes measured in the same way for all groups?	☐	☐	☐	☐
9. Were outcomes measured in a reliable way?	☐	☐	☐	☐
10. Are reports of the study free of suggestion of selective outcome reporting?	☐	☐	☐	☐

(Higgins and Green 2008; Guyatt et al. 2015; Joanna Briggs Institute 2014)

Assessing Observational Studies

A wide range of study designs can be subsumed under the category "observational studies." This type of study evaluates the effect of an intervention, but no randomized assignment of participants takes place. The category includes controlled and uncontrolled studies such as nonrandomized studies, controlled before-and-after studies, time series studies, cohort studies, case control studies, and case series. Definitions or descriptions of various study designs can be found on glossary websites from the Online Learning Center of McGraw-Hill or the Cochrane Community from the Cochrane Collaboration (see appendix at end of chapter). Incorporating the evidence from observational studies in a review may address gaps in the evidence from randomized studies on the effects of interventions (Morton et al. 2011). Furthermore, there may be only observational studies available to address certain research questions of harm, etiology, or prognosis in clinical research, or questions on effectiveness of educational interventions on learning outcomes.

The quality criteria used to judge the internal validity in randomized trials allow for an overall quality assessment of objective aspects of study methods and cover major threats or risks of bias. The criteria may be applied to carry out a minimum assessment review of observational studies. However, not all criteria for randomized studies may be suitable for observational studies with various designs. For example, in assessing studies of prognosis, the quality assessment item of randomization may not be appropriate; instead, the assessment should look at the similarity of comparison groups at baseline regarding prognostic factors and the percent of follow-up (Glasziou 2001). For case control studies, they are likely prone to recall bias in which cases may be more likely to recall potential risk factors for the outcome in question. One way to avoid such bias is to use a standardized instrument (e.g., questionnaire) to elicit information from cases and controls; the interviewer who administers the questionnaire is blind to whether the interviewee is a case or control (Petticrew and Roberts 2006).

Observational studies with different characteristics and design methods may be subject to a wide variability of biases and the between-study heterogeneity inherent in study designs. The methodological diversity of these studies included for a review may lead to variations between studies in their risk of selection bias, variations in how confounding factors are controlled in the study design and implementation, or even greater risk of other biases resulting from poor design and execution. Due to the methodological diversity and extra sources of bias in observational studies, they are more heterogeneous than randomized studies. Since there is no single best tool for assessing observational studies, reviewers may need to use additional quality assessment items or create several tools for assessment of risk of bias in studies with different design features. In using additional quality assessment items or supplementary instruments, reviewers need to consider how adequately confounding was dealt with in observational studies (Egger, Altman, and Schneider 2008) and whether assessment tools have been used previously and validated or checked for reliability. Furthermore, reviewers are cautioned against using meta-analysis to combine effect estimates of randomized trials with those of nonrandomized studies or across nonrandomized studies with different designs. Having reviewers with deeper knowledge of epidemiology or research methods on the review team would be of great value to the critical appraisal process because they can help identify possible pitfalls or key areas of weakness in included studies with diverse designs (Higgins and Green 2008).

The appendix lists several risks of bias assessment tools that may be used to guide the process in critical appraisal of observational studies. In using any of the tools, reviewers may need to modify a tool of their choice or add specific assessment items to fit in with their review questions. Given the subjective nature of an individual reviewer's interpretation and rating of assessment criteria, an assessment tool needs to be pilot tested with a sample of full-text articles to ensure its appropriateness and relevance for critical appraisal of included studies in a review.

Assessing Cross-Sectional Studies

In a cross-sectional study, researchers survey a group of people or a representative sample at just one point in time. This type of study design is commonly used in medical research, educational research, social science, and other fields of research. Cross-sectional research design is increasingly included in reviews of effectiveness of interventions. A questionnaire is often used as a survey tool to collect a range of different types of data (both quantitative and qualitative data) about people's knowledge, beliefs, attitudes, and behaviors and to answer questions of what, how, and why. Although it appears easy to write up a list of questions (or items) and to ask people to respond, a cross-sectional study with a poorly written questionnaire can lead to spurious data, misleading conclusions, and nebulous recommendations (Greenhalgh 2010). There are abundant tools and guides that have been developed and validated for assessing randomized studies, but few comparable assessment tools are available for survey research. Box 8.4 presents a framework for appraising surveys by drawing upon several existing guides (Crombie 1996; Greenhalgh 2005). Reviewers may use the framework as a basis and add additional assessment items in critical appraisal of cross-sectional studies or studies using mixed research methods. Speaking of the evidence collected from a survey,

Roger Jowell voiced this view: "Every finding is an approximation, part of a body of evidence which needs to be examined in the context of other evidence" (Jowell 1984). As reviewers, bear in mind that no finding from a survey can be taken as a definitive or precise statement about a person's own attitude or thinking mind.

TEXTBOX 8.4. CHECKLIST FOR APPRAISING SURVEYS

Quality indicators	*Yes*	*No*	*Unclear*	*N/A*
1. Did the study address a clearly focused research question?	☐	☐	☐	☐
2. Is the research method (study design) appropriate for answering the research question?	☐	☐	☐	☐
3. Is the method of selection of participants (patients, students, faculty, customers) clearly described?	☐	☐	☐	☐
4. Is the sample of participants representative with regard to the population to which the findings will be generalized?	☐	☐	☐	☐
5. Could the way the sample was obtained introduce potential (selection) bias?	☐	☐	☐	☐
6. Was a pilot version of a survey administered to participants representative of those in the sampling frame, and the instrument modified accordingly?	☐	☐	☐	☐
7. Was the survey used in the study likely to be valid and reliable?	☐	☐	☐	☐
8. If the study compares different subgroups from the survey, were the data obtained using the same methods from these different groups?	☐	☐	☐	☐
9. Was the response rate adequate?	☐	☐	☐	☐
10. Have nonresponders been accounted for?	☐	☐	☐	☐
11. Was the statistical analysis appropriate (e.g., statistical analysis for quantitative answers, qualitative analysis for open-ended questions)?				
12. Is there an adequate description of the data?	☐	☐	☐	☐
13. Have all relevant results ("significant" and "nonsignificant") been reported?	☐	☐	☐	☐

(Greenhalgh 2005; Greenhalgh 2010; Petticrew and Roberts 2006)

LIBRARIAN PARTICIPATION IN CRITICAL APPRAISAL

Librarians can be at the forefront of the critical appraisal of included studies in a systematic review from the inception of the study selection process. Their roles in a systematic review need not be confined to conducting literature searches or methodology write-up. In addition to their involvement in the citation and study screening process, they can contribute to critical appraisal in various ways as described in librarian's corner 8.2.

Librarian's Corner 8.2: Librarian Roles in Critical Appraisal

- Identifying and selecting an appropriate assessment tool and pilot testing the tool with a sample of selected studies
- Serving as peer reviewer in pilot testing a selected assessment tool and in performing the critical appraisal task
- Functioning as an arbitrator or tiebreaker to help resolve any disagreement in judgments between reviewers
- Managing paper audit trails associated with the consistent use of assessment criteria and evaluation of individual studies to ensure a systematic, transparent, and reproducible procedure
- Communicating with original authors of selected studies for clarification of study methods and procurement of unreported outcome data and other detailed information on selected studies if needed
- Taking the lead for project management of the review process and keeping the review team on task
- Consulting in critical appraisal and providing training opportunities to educate researchers about the critical appraisal process

The level of librarian involvement in critical appraisal is influential to the conduct and end result of a systematic review because of their expertise, perspectives, information management and evaluation skills, and their ability to interact and communicate with researchers across disciplines and research fields. Promoting and advocating the important role for librarians in critical appraisal and other parts of the review process are likely to help enhance the quality of a review and in turn expand library services and propel librarians' professional development for sustaining their vitality (Mi 2016).

CONCLUSION

Extensive discussion and explication of critical appraisal of studies of various research designs and existing quality assessment tools are beyond the scope of this chapter. It is an attempt of the chapter to provide an introduction to the general practice in the process of study selection and critical appraisal in a systematic review. The increased demand for and wide use of research synthesis for evidence-based decision making in health care and other sectors have created a window of opportunity for libraries to reinvent traditional library services and information literacy instruction programs. Librarians' roles and contributions to a systematic review related to study selection and critical appraisal are conspicuous and influential to effective design, conduct, and reporting of a systematic review.

APPENDIX: SELECTION AND CRITICAL APPRAISAL TOOLS

Tool for Judging the Body of Evidence as a Whole		
GRADE Approach	Neumann, I., N. Santesso, E. A. Akl, D. M. Rind, P. O. Vandvik, P. Alonso-Coello, T. Agoritsas, R. Mustafa, P. E. Alexander, H. Schunemann, and G. H. Guyatt. 2016. "A Guide for Health Professionals to Interpret and Use Recommendations in Guidelines Developed with the GRADE Approach." *Journal of Clinical Epidemiology*. doi:10.1016/j.jclinepi.2015.11.017.	http://www.ncbi.nlm.nih.gov/pubmed/26772609
Tools for Assessing Randomized Studies		
Assessment of Multiple Systematic Reviews (AMSTAR)	Shea, B. J., J. M. Grimshaw, G. A. Wells, M. Boers, N. Andersson, C. Hamel, A. C. Porter, P. Tugwell, D. Moher, and L. M. Bouter. 2007. "Development of	http://amstar.ca/Amstar_Checklist.php

	AMSTAR: A Measurement Tool to Assess the Methodological Quality of Systematic Reviews." *BMC Medical Research Methodology* 7:10. doi:10.1186/1471-2288-7-10.	
CASP Randomized Controlled Trial Checklist	The Critical Appraisal Skills Programme (CASP)	http://tinyurl.com/zwqqugy
Tools for Assessing Observational Studies		
Analysis Manual: Steps in the Academy Evidence Analysis Process	Academy of Nutrition and Dietetics	http://tinyurl.com/z6sy9ym
CASP Cohort Study Checklist	The Critical Appraisal Skills Programme (CASP)	http://tinyurl.com/gub25e7
CASP Case Control Checklist	The Critical Appraisal Skills Programme (CASP)	http://tinyurl.com/pmujmu2
Guide to scoring methods using the Maryland Scientific Methods Scale	What Works Centre for Local Economic Growth	http://www.whatworksgrowth.org/public/files/Scoring-Guide.pdf
Interrupted time series (ITS) analyses	Cochrane Effective Practice and Organizational Care (EPOC group)	http://tinyurl.com/zu6wnog
STROBE Checklist (Strengthening the reporting of observational studies in epidemiology)	von Elm, E., G. Poglia, B. Walder, and M. R. Tramer. 2004. "Different Patterns of Duplicate Publication: An Analysis of Articles Used in Systematic Reviews." *JAMA* 291 (8): 974–80. doi:10.1001/jama.291.8.974.	http://www.ncbi.nlm.nih.gov/pubmed/18064739
Transparent Reporting of Evaluations with Nonrandomized Designs (TREND) statement	Des Jarlais, D. C., C. Lyles, and N. Crepaz. 2004. "Improving the Reporting Quality of Nonrandomized Evaluations of Behavioral and Public Health	http://www.ncbi.nlm.nih.gov/pubmed/?term=14998794

	Interventions: The TREND Statement." *American Journal of Public Health* 94 (3): 361–66.	
Tools for Assessing Qualitative Studies		
10 Questions to Help You Make Sense of Qualitative Research	Critical Appraisal Skills Programme (CASP)	http://tinyurl.com/m4kbv7f
EPPI-Centre Methods for Conducting Systematic Reviews	Evidence for Policy and Practice Information and Co-ordinating Centre (EPPI-Centre)	http://tinyurl.com/zwp976k
Evaluation Tool for Quantitative Research Studies	Long, Andrew, and Mary Godfrey. 2004. "An Evaluation Tool to Assess the Quality of Qualitative Research Studies." *International Journal of Social Research Methodology* 7 (2): 181–96.	http://usir.salford.ac.uk/12969
Guidelines for Critical Review Form: Qualitative Studies (Version 2.0)	McMaster University School of Rehabilitation Science	http://tinyurl.com/hzqh5q8
Joanna Briggs Institute Reviewers' Manual 2014 Edition	The Joanna Briggs Institute	http://www.joannabriggs.org/assets/docs/sumari/ReviewersManual_2014-The-Systematic-Review-of-Prevalence-and-Incidence-Data_v2.pdf
Quality in Qualitative Evaluation: A Framework for Assessing Research Evidence	Liz Spencer, Jane Ritchie, Jane Lewis, and Lucy Dillon from the National Centre for Social Research in the UK	http://tinyurl.com/hgkxzlp
Tools for Assessing Mixed Methods Research		
A Scoring System for Appraising Mixed Methods Research	Pluye, P., M. P. Gagnon, F. Griffiths, and J. Johnson-Lafleur. 2009. "A Scoring System for Appraising Mixed Methods Research, and Concomitantly Appraising	http://www.ncbi.nlm.nih.gov/pubmed/19233357

	Qualitative, Quantitative and Mixed Methods Primary Studies in Mixed Studies Reviews." *International Journal of Nursing Studies* 46 (4): 529–46.	
Evaluation Tool for Mixed Methods Studies	Long, A. F., M. Godfrey, T. Randall, A. J. Brettle, and M. J. Grant. 2002. "Developing Evidence Based Social Care Policy and Practice. Part 3: Feasibility of Undertaking Systematic Reviews in Social Care." Leeds: Nuffield Institute for Health	http://usir.salford.ac.uk/13070
Glossary		
Name	Source	Web Address
Glossary	JAMAevidence	http://jamaevidence.mhmedical.com/glossary.aspx
Cochrane Community Glossary	The Cochrane Collaboration	https://community.cochrane.org/glossary
Online Learning Center	Fraenkel, Jack R., Norman E. Wallen, and Helen H. Hyun. 2011. *How to Design and Evaluate Research in Education*. 8th ed. New York: McGraw-Hill Humanities/Social Sciences/Languages.	http://highered.mheducation.com/sites/0072532491/student_view0/glossary.html

REFERENCES

Boland, Angela, G. Cherry, and R. Dickson. 2014. *Doing a Systematic Review*. Los Angeles: Sage.

Booth, Andrew, Diana Papaioannou, and Anthea Sutton. 2012. *Systematic Approaches to a Successful Literature Review*. Los Angeles: Sage.

Cooper, H. M. 2010. "Research Synthesis and Meta-Analysis: A Step-by-Step Approach." In *Applied Social Research Methods Series*, 4th ed. Los Angeles: Sage.

Crombie, Iain Kinloch. 1996. *The Pocket Guide to Critical Appraisal*. London: BMJ Publishing Group.

Egger, Matthias, Douglas Altman, and M. Schneider. 2008. "Systematic Review of Observational Studies." In *Systematic Reviews in Health Care Meta-Analysis in Context*, 211–27. London: BMJ Books.

Gall, Meredith D., Walter R. Borg, and Joyce P. Gall. 2007. *Educational Research*. 8th ed. Boston: Pearson/Allyn & Bacon.

Garg, Amit X., Dan Hackam, and Marcello Tonelli. 2008. "Systematic Review and Meta-Analysis: When One Study Is Just Not Enough." *Clinical Journal of the American Society of Nephrology* 3 (1): 253–60. doi:10.2215/CJN.01430307. http://cjasn.asnjournals.org/content/3/1/253.

Glasziou, Paul. 2001. *Systematic Reviews in Health Care: A Practical Guide*. Cambridge: Cambridge University Press. http://lib.myilibrary.com?ID=16222.

Gough, David, Sandy Oliver, and James Thomas. 2012. *Introduction to Systematic Reviews*. Los Angeles: Sage.

Greenhalgh, Trisha. 2005. *Diffusion of Innovations in Health Service Organisations: A Systematic Literature Review*. New York: McGraw-Hill Education.

Greenhalgh, Trisha. 2010. *How to Read a Paper*. 4th ed. Hoboken, NJ: Wiley-Blackwell.

Haase, Steven C. 2011. "Systematic Reviews and Meta-Analysis." *Plastic and Reconstructive Surgery* 127 (2): 955–66. doi:10.1097/PRS.0b013e318200afa9. http://www.ncbi.nlm.nih.gov/pubmed/clipboard.

Herbison, Peter, Jean Hay-Smith, and William J. Gillespie. 2006. "Adjustment of Meta-Analyses on the Basis of Quality Scores Should Be Abandoned." *Journal of Clinical Epidemiology* 59 (12): 1249–56. doi:10.1016/j.jclinepi.2006.03.008. http://www.ncbi.nlm.nih.gov/pubmed/clipboard.

Higgins, Julian P. T., Sally Green, and Cochrane Collaboration. 2008. *Cochrane Handbook for Systematic Reviews of Interventions*. Chichester, England; Hoboken, NJ: Wiley-Blackwell.

Institute of Medicine. 2010. *Finding What Works in Health Care*. Washington, DC: National Academies Press.

The Joanna Briggs Institute. 2016. Joanna Briggs Institute Reviewers' Manual: 2016 edition. Australia: The Joanna Briggs Institute.

Jowell, Roger. 1984. "Introducing the Survey." In *British Social Attitudes: The 1984 Report*, ed. R. Jowell and C. Airey, 1–10. Aldershot, UK: Gower.

Jüni, P., A. Witschi, R. Bloch, and M. Egger. 1999. "The Hazards of Scoring the Quality of Clinical Trials for Meta-Analysis." *JAMA* 282 (11): 1054–60. http://www.ncbi.nlm.nih.gov/pubmed/clipboard.

Khan, K. S., S. Daya, and A. Jadad. 1996. "The Importance of Quality of Primary Studies in Producing Unbiased Systematic Reviews." *Archives of Internal Medicine* 156 (6): 661–66. http://www.ncbi.nlm.nih.gov/pubmed/clipboard.

Khan, Khalid, Regina Kunz, Jos Kleijnen, and Gerd Antes. 2011. *Systematic Reviews to Support Evidence-Based Medicine*. 2nd ed. Boca Raton, FL: CRC Press.

Liberati, A., D. G. Altman, J. Tetzlaff, C. Mulrow, P. C. Gøtzsche, et al. 2009. "The PRISMA Statement for Reporting Systematic Reviews and Meta-Analyses of

Studies That Evaluate Health Care Interventions: Explanation and Elaboration." *PLoS Medicine* 6 (7): e1000100. doi:10.1371/journal.pmed.1000100.

Littell, Julia H., Jacqueline Corcoran, and Vijayan K. Pillai. 2008. *Systematic Reviews and Meta-Analysis, Pocket Guides to Social Work Research Methods*. New York: Oxford University Press.

Marchevsky, Alberto M., and Mark R. Wick. 2011. *Evidence Based Pathology and Laboratory Medicine*. New York: Springer. doi:10.1007/978-1-4419-1030-1.

Mi, M. 2016. "Leveraging Research Synthesis for Promoting and Expanding Library Services and Educational Programs." *Journal of Academic Librarianship* 42 (2): 151–53.

Moher, D., A. R. Jadad, G. Nichol, M. Penman, P. Tugwell, and S. Walsh. 1995. "Assessing the Quality of Randomized Controlled Trials: An Annotated Bibliography of Scales and Checklists." *Controlled Clinical Trials* 16 (1): 62–73.

Moher, D., A. R. Jadad, and P. Tugwell. 1996. "Assessing the Quality of Randomized Controlled Trials: Current Issues and Future Directions." *International Journal of Technology Assessment in Health Care* 12 (2): 195–208.

Morton, Sally, Laura Levit, Alfred Berg, and Jill Eden. 2011. *Finding What Works in Health Care: Standards for Systematic Reviews*. Washington, DC: National Academies Press.

Nelson, Heidi D. 2014. *Systematic Reviews to Answer Health Care Questions*. Philadelphia, PA: Wolters Kluwer Health.

Pearson, Alan, John Field, and Zoe Jordan. 2009. *Evidence-Based Clinical Practice in Nursing and Health Care: Assimilating Research, Experience and Expertise*. Malden, MA: Wiley.

Petticrew, Mark, and Helen Roberts. 2006. *Systematic Reviews in the Social Sciences: A Practical Guide*. Malden, MA: Blackwell Publishers.

Shadish, William, and David Myers. 2004. "Research Design Policy Brief." Accessed January 16, 2016. http://www.campbellcollaboration.org/artman2/uploads/1/C2_Research_Design_Policy_Brief-2.pdf.

Smith, M. L. 1980. "Publication Bias and Meta-Analysis." *Evaluation in Education* 4: 22–24.

Tramer, M. R., D. J. Reynolds, R. A. Moore, and H. J. McQuay. 1997. "Impact of Covert Duplicate Publication on Meta-Analysis: A Case Study." *BMJ* 315 (7109): 635–40.

Wongpakaran, Nahathai, Tinakon Wongpakaran, Danny Wedding, and Kilem L. Gwet. 2013. "A Comparison of Cohen's Kappa and Gwet's AC1 When Calculating Inter-Rater Reliability Coefficients: A Study Conducted with Personality Disorder Samples." *BMC Medical Research Methodology* 13:61. doi:10.1186/1471-2288-13-61.

Chapter Nine

Collecting and Combining Study Data and Explaining the Findings

Margaret J. Foster

We are approaching a new age of synthesis. Knowledge cannot be merely a degree or a skill . . . it demands a broader vision, capabilities in critical thinking and logical deduction without which we cannot have constructive progress.

—Li Ka-shing

OBJECTIVES

- Describe the data collection and synthesis process
- List the standards for conducting this step and reporting methods
- Describe processes for quality assurance
- Detail the potential involvement of the librarian

OVERVIEW

Collecting and synthesizing the included studies' data, as well as explaining and contextualizing the findings are what the review authors originally set out to do. Although the steps leading up to this step are required, they are just a precursor for the synthesis. Data collection is at the "core of a systematic review because accurate data and their synthesis form the basis of appropriate conclusions" (Li et al. 2015, 287). It is the most time consuming and difficult part of the process, but also the most rewarding as the review authors finally get to wrestle with the studies in which they are most interested and end with answering their research question. This chapter introduces the process of data abstraction and synthesis, while emphasizing the need for quality practices.

Well-designed data collection methods should be comprehensive, accurate, and transparent (Li et al. 2015). While most librarians will not fully participate in this step, it is important to understand the overall process to determine potential ways to support or collaborate on this step. There are five main steps for this stage of the review, as listed in box 9.1.

TEXTBOX 9.1. SUGGESTED STEPS FOR COLLECTING AND COMBINING DATA

Step 1: Plan synthesis
Step 2: List data elements
Step 3: Develop data collection methods
Step 4: Develop form and collect data
Step 5: Complete synthesis and explain the findings

LIBRARIAN'S CORNER 9.1. LIBRARIAN ROLES IN COLLECTING AND COMBINING STUDY DATA AND EXPLAINING THE SYNTHESIS

- Provide resources that describe how to select and conduct synthesis techniques
- Provide links to potential software tools for data collection/synthesis and/or subscribe to online resources
- Provide examples of data elements
- Provide examples of existing forms
- Help obtain unpublished data

STEP 1: SELECT TYPES OF SYNTHESIS

Before listing the data elements to be abstracted, it is important to consider the different types of synthesis that could be conducted. The types of synthesis are not exclusive, as one review can include more than one type of synthesis. No matter the specific type(s) of syntheses selected, there is a similar set of processes review authors need to complete. During the planning stage, authors should consider four factors when selecting an appropriate synthesis method:

- What is the specificity of the review's objective—is it exploratory or very specific?
- What type of studies are being included?
- What are the resources available to the team, including expertise on synthesis?
- Has a framework been established for the topic being reviewed?

The methods of how to select a synthesis continue to evolve, especially concerning how to synthesize information qualitatively. A framework depicts the relationships between stakeholders, variables, concepts, and/or other factors within a particular phenomenon (Gough, Oliver, and Thomas 2012). Reviews of effectiveness are designed around a specific question which provides the framework—what interventions work for a particular population? Some methodologists have called for systematic review authors to include a logic model in the protocol and/or report of the review. A logic model is an extension of the conceptual framework and is "a summary diagram which maps out an intervention and conjectured links between the intervention and anticipated outcomes in order to develop a summarised theory of how a complex intervention works" (Baxter et al. 2014). Kneale, Thomas, and Harris

Table 9.1. Guidance on synthesis methods

Topic	*Resources*
Selecting synthesis type	Kastner et al. 2016. Conceptual recommendations for selecting the most appropriate knowledge synthesis method to answer research questions related to complex evidence
	Booth et al. 2016. Guidance on choosing qualitative evidence synthesis methods for use in health technology assessments of complex interventions
Narrative synthesis	Snilstveit et al. 2012. Narrative approaches to systematic review and synthesis of evidence for international development policy and practice
Quantitative synthesis	Field and Gillet 2010. How to do a meta-analysis
Integrative synthesis	Pluye 2015. Mixed kinds of evidence: synthesis designs and critical appraisal for systematic mixed studies reviews including qualitative, quantitative, and mixed methods studies
	Heyvaert et al. 2013. Mixed methods research synthesis: definition, framework, and potential

published a step-by-step guide on how to develop a logic model for systematic reviews (Kneale, Thomas, and Harris 2015). Other types of reviews are attempting to develop a framework. Table 9.1 provides a list of resources to help in selecting which synthesis type to conduct as well as guides on various types of synthesis. The following sections describe a range of synthesis types.

Qualitative Synthesis Methods

Narrative Synthesis

The most common approach is narrative synthesis, which can be used with any type of study and in almost every systematic review alongside other synthesis techniques. It is usually the first step in analyzing and organizing the data and generally involves summarizing multiple studies with text and can be utilized with any type of data. Narrative synthesis can be difficult as there has been little written to guide or standardize the process (Rodgers et al. 2009). In addition, reviews with a high number of studies, studies that vary greatly in design and other characteristics, or studies that explore/examine complex questions are difficult to summarize. Despite the challenges, the synthesis methods should be rigorous, transparent, systematic, and specified in the methods. Table 9.2 provides a brief list of potential techniques.

Qualitative Synthesis of Qualitative Studies

Authors of reviews including qualitative studies may need to select other types of qualitative techniques. The selection will depend on whether a conceptual framework exists. To develop a framework, authors may select grounded theory, meta-ethnography, or a thematic synthesis. A framework synthesis may be appropriate if a framework already exists, but authors want the flexibility to adapt it based on review (Gough, Oliver, and Thomas 2012). A variant of this type is called the best fit framework analysis, "which may be very helpful when policymakers, practitioners or other decision makers need answers quickly, and are able to tolerate some ambiguity about whether the answer is the very best that could be given" (Dixon-Woods 2011). It is important to note that thematic and framework synthesis cannot also be used on quantitative studies (Gough, Thomas, and Oliver 2012).

Quantitative Synthesis Methods

Meta-analyses are one of the rarest forms of synthesis, as the set of criteria for when it is appropriate to conduct this synthesis is rarely met. First, consider if

Table 9.2. Narrative synthesis techniques

Technique	*Description*	*Advantage*	*Limitation*
Text description	Consistent annotation of studies: organized summary of same characteristics	Keeps details of each study together	Difficult to see themes
Tabulation	Create table of study elements and findings	Compare characteristics	Does not synthesize
Categorize	Group or cluster studies around particular characteristic(s)	Visualize patterns	May limit the ability to see concepts across all studies
Thematic analysis	Content analysis with a rubric to identify themes and factors	Consistency	Takes time to develop the rubric
Describe relationships	Relationships between primary study findings and characteristics of study Determine differences within and between studies	Provides subanalysis	May be difficult with a large number of studies

Source: Booth, Papaioannou, and Sutton 2012

Table 9.3. Software for qualitative synthesis

Software	*Developer*	*Link*	*Cost?*
ATLAS.ti	ATLAS.ti Scientific Software Development	www.atlasti.de	Yes
EPPI-Reviewer	EPPI Centre, Institute of Education, University of London	eppi.ioe.ac.uk	Yes
MAXQDA	VERBI	http://www.maxqda.com	Yes
Nvivo	QSR International	www.qsrinternational.com	Yes
QARI	Joanna Briggs Institute	www.joannabriggs.edu	No
Qualitative Data Analysis Program (QDAP)	University of Massachusetts Amherst	http://www.umass.edu/qdap	No

it is appropriate to combine the studies together. While heterogeneity will be calculated to determine the statistical appropriateness of meta-analysis, it is also important that studies are logically similar. Second, consider the goal of the synthesis. If the goal is to report a summary effect, then multiple variables of the studies should be similar (populations, interventions, and other relevant characteristics). However, if the goal is to demonstrate the variety of effects due to a confounding factor, then all relevant studies should be included. Including studies with minor differences could be handled in analysis, but having too few studies could present issues (Borenstein et al. 2009). Researchers considering a meta-analysis without experience should consider consulting an expert. Table 9.4 lists potential meta-analysis software.

Table 9.4. Software for meta-analysis

Resource	*Developer*	*Link*	*Cost*
Comprehensive Meta-Analysis (CMA)	Biostat Inc.	https://www.meta-analysis.com	Yes
Mix 2.0	Biostatxl	http://www.meta-analysis-made-easy.com	Free lite version available
OpenMeta[Analyst]	Brown University	http://www.cebm.brown.edu/openmeta	No

Integrative-Combining Quantitative and Qualitative Synthesis Techniques

There are several types of reviews which combine both quantitative and qualitative studies in addition to narrative reviews previously described. While meta-analysis calculates a combined effect size of quantitative studies, a qualitative synthesis of quantitative or qualitative studies helps to identify and provide additional information about the effect size. A Bayesian meta-synthesis that combines both types of studies will therefore "more properly reflect the diversity of evidence at primary level," providing a richer source of evidence for decision making (Kastner et al. 2016). Realist synthesis or review goes beyond the typical "what works" review to answer "why, for whom, and in what context" and combines theoretical, qualitative, and quantitative studies to decide if the current theories match the evidence or need to be modified (Booth, Papaioannou, and Sutton 2012). Mixed methods review is a "synthesis in which researchers combine qualitative, quantitative, and mixed methods studies, and apply a mixed methods approach in order to integrate those studies, for the broad purposes of breadth and depth of understanding and corroboration" (Heyvaert, Maes, and Onghena 2013).

STEP 2: DATA ELEMENTS

List and Group Data Elements

The data elements to extract from each study will depend on the objective(s) of the review, the type of question the review is aiming to answer, and the types of studies. For instance, for studies that include some type of participant, one set of elements would be study participant characteristics, such as age, gender, grade level in school, or sociodemographics. After items have been listed, group the data elements in groups or in order of where the element is expected to appear in the study reports. Table 9.5 lists data elements grouped by topics, gathered from a variety of reporting standards for primary studies such as STARD or CONSORT, and by guidelines for conducting reviews such as the *Cochrane Handbook*. The Cochrane Collaboration provides a list of data elements (see *Cochrane Handbook*, table 7.3a) for intervention studies and is a great starting point for those coding these types of studies (Higgins, Green, and Cochrane Collaboration 2008). For other types of studies, these data elements may not be necessary or appropriate.

Table 9.5. Potential data elements

Category	*Examples of elements*
Participants	Number of participants, age, gender, sociodemographics, race/ethnicity, diagnostic criteria
Method	Study design (randomization methods, masking), number of study arms, study/intervention implementers, training for implementation, setting, geography, study duration
Results	Time points, number of participants who completed the study, summary data for each group, estimate effects with confidence intervals; p-value; adverse effects
Other	Funding source, application of findings, authors' conclusions

Source: Jonnalagadda, Goyal, and Huffman 2015

For Each Data Element, Determine How to Best Collect the Data

Consider each element and whether it will have open coding or categorical coding. If a data element has a known or prespecified set of possible categories or choices, then these categories need to be clearly defined and tested to ensure that coders use them consistently. Other elements may need to be open coded, as it is unknown what the possible categories are for these characteristics. It is important to code each data element in a way that is most effective for completing the review and for utilizing the data afterward. For example, if there are many studies to code, having several open coding questions will be very time consuming to synthesize afterward.

Draft Evidence Tables and Figures

Drafting potential tables and figures that are expected to be produced from the data elements is a useful activity, in that review authors will begin to best envision how the results of coding will be utilized. Sometimes it will reveal that there are some data elements that are not necessary or some that have been missed. In addition, it will help in developing the form, as it can be done in such a way that the tables are easier to create.

STEP 3: DEVELOP DATA COLLECTION METHODS

Now that a list of data elements has been established, consider how the data collection will be conducted, including number of coders, division of articles, quality assurance, and software.

Selecting Coders and Planning Disagreement Resolution

The review authors will need to decide who will code, including if additional coders are needed. In 2010, Horton et al. considered the experience of authors in data collection and if this affected accuracy. Their findings highlighted that the number of errors remained the same; however, time to complete was different, with less experienced coders taking much more time to complete. While familiarity with the topic is important, accurate data collection also needs "adequate instruction, training and care" (Horton et al. 2010). One of the standards for systematic reviews that can cause hardships is the call for double data abstraction or data collection by two independent coders. Research has shown that this standard is important as single extraction leads to more mistakes than double extraction (Buscemi et al. 2006). AMSTAR and other evaluative checklists of systematic reviews rate reviews higher for having done this. If each study is independently coded, then disagreements are likely to occur. The review team needs to determine how those differences will be found and resolved—such as by consensus of the pair, the entire team, or a third coder.

Missing or Vague Data

When pulling information from studies, some details of the study may not be easy to collect or code because the information is missing, vague, or cannot be discerned from a graph or figure. The review author(s) need to strategize how these situations are going to be handled. Will primary study authors be contacted? Will data from graphs/figures be estimated or will actual data be required/requested? Some methodologists have proposed having coders use a scale to express their confidence in the information. This is especially true of vital data, such as effect sizes (Wilson 2009).

Select a Tool

When selecting a data tool, clients should evaluate the tool's availability, usability, cost, training, and support (see table 4.6 in chapter 4). In addition, consider data curation and sharing options for future use, as some tools, such as Systematic Review Data Repository (SRDR), make it easier to share with others. Table 9.6 has a list of potential tools ranging from paper and pen to complex data repositories.

STEP 4: DEVELOP FORM AND COLLECT DATA

Develop the Form and Train Coders

Use the list created during step 2 to develop the form in the selected software. It is also important to consider that studies are being coded, not articles, so that if one study is described in multiple articles, it will need to be coded only once. The form needs to be tested by considering the range of studies from the sample to be coded and testing studies representing the sample (Cooper 2009). One method for training is to have testers on the team fill out the form using the same set of studies, then discuss the issues. If there is a large team of coders, a codebook may be appropriate, which is a document detailing how to fill in each data element. The codebook is also useful to add to data archives about the coding forms to ease understanding.

Data Collection

During the data collection process, it is important to employ quality control practices to ensure accurate and complete data collection. The review team should assign someone to ensure that the process runs smoothly. Bias could be introduced during coding if the reviewer codes studies differently due to the nature of its findings, authors, journal title, or other aspects of the study. To overcome this, many standards, such as AMSTAR, call for having each study extracted independently by two reviewers (Shea et al. 2007).

Table 9.6. Potential data collection tools

Format	*Examples*	*Advantages*	*Disadvantages*
Paper forms	Create form in Microsoft Word, Google Docs, or other word processor and print	• Quick to create • Requires few resources • Easy to determine if form is complete • Does not require a computer or network connectivity	• Information will need to be typed into appropriate software at some point leading to inefficiency or potential for mistakes • Difficulty increases with number of studies to code
Databases	Microsoft Access	• Can specify data format • Save data as they work (reduces chance of data loss) • Data can often be exported to stat. software (depends)	• High learning curve • Cost • Time
Spreadsheet	Microsoft Excel, Google Sheets, FileMaker Pro	• Quick to create • Low learning curve	• Corrupted data
Forms	Adobe Acrobat, Google Forms, Qualtrics, Survey Monkey	• Relatively low learning curve	• Need to track if an article was completed outside of the software
Review specific software	Covidence, Systematic Review Data Repository, Distiller	• Designed to meet needs of reviewers • Can provide data curation	• High learning curve • Cost

Sources: Cooper et al. 2014; Li et al. 2015

STEP 5: SYNTHESIZING AND EXPLAINING THE FINDINGS

The main goal of the synthesis is to answer the main question or objective of the review. Once the studies are coded, authors summarize the results with text, tables, and figures and explain the meaning of the results. Readers of reviews need enough details about the included studies to decide if the results can apply to a particular situation. If the studies focused on participants in some way, the overall demographics and important characteristics of those participants should be provided. The methodological standards for the conduct of new Cochrane Intervention Reviews list what should be included in a summary table in standard C75 (Chandler et al. 2013).

In addition to the summary of the studies' characteristics, review authors should address the overall quality of the studies. Grading of Recommendations Assessment, Development, and Evaluation (GRADE) offers guidance on how to do this with clinical topics and is one of the most widely used systems. It calls for review authors to consider five issues (study limitations, consistency of effect, imprecision, indirectness, and publication bias) when evaluating the overall quality of evidence (Mao et al. 2013). The CERQuaL framework (stands for Confidence in the Evidence from Reviews of Qualitative research) was developed for synthesizing evidence quality for qualitative research (Lewin et al. 2015). Table 9.7 provides resources to assist with this step.

Of particular interest to librarians will be the potential for publication bias, which can result from a limited search. Publication bias is a group of biases (location bias, database bias, language bias) which lead to studies not being published as widely due to the nature of the findings (in other words, the findings are influencing the likelihood that a study is published). A 2016 report evaluated over 1,100 systematic reviews from the Cochrane Library and found that if a primary study had an outcome favoring treatment, it was 27 percent more likely to be published (Kicinski, Springate, and Kontopantelis 2015). Publication bias can only be measured mathematically if a meta-analysis is conducted; otherwise, it can only be described in the narrative, describing the likelihood that studies were missed. Booth et al. (2016) provides calls for review authors to consider the following factors in regard to grey literature and/or non-English studies:

- Did the databases/sources searched cover these publications?
- Were these publications represented in the included studies?
- If non-English language studies were excluded, can it be determined from the English abstract the direction of the outcome? Was the direction similar to included studies?

If a meta-analysis was conducted, then a funnel plot can be produced to visually demonstrate the risk of publication bias.

Finally, the review authors need to analyze the results and place the findings into context. (Box 9.2 details the questions that need to be answered.) Throughout this process, review authors are encouraged to consider the

Table 9.7. Guides for synthesizing appraisal of the evidence

Approach	*Developer*	*Designed for*	*Reference*
Evidence-based Practice Center (EPC) approach	Agency for Healthcare Research and Quality (AHRQ)	RCTs and observational trials	1
C2 Checklist for Assessment of Methodological Quality in Economic Evaluation Studies	Campbell Collaboration	Quantitative economic evaluations	2
GRADE	Cochrane Collaboration	Randomized control trials	3
CERQuaL (Confidence in the Evidence from Reviews of Qualitative Research)	GRADE Working Group	Qualitative studies in clinical health	4
FAME (Feasibility, Appropriateness, Meaningfulness, Effectiveness)	Joanna Briggs Institute (JBI)	Qualitative and quantitative	5

Sources (as numbered above):

1. N. D. Berkman, K. N. Lohr, M. Ansari, M. McDonagh, E. Balk, E. Whitlock, J. Reston, E. Bass, M. Butler, G. Gartlehner, L. Hartling, R. Kane, M. McPheeters, L. Morgan, S. C. Morton, M. Viswanathan, P. Sista, and S. Chang, "Grading the Strength of a Body of Evidence When Assessing Health Care Interventions for the Effective Health Care Program of the Agency for Healthcare Research and Quality: An Update," in *Methods Guide for Comparative Effectiveness Reviews* (Rockville, MD: Agency for Healthcare Research and Quality: 2013), 4, http://effectivehealthcare.ahrq.gov/ehc/products/457/1752/methodsguidance-grading-evidence-131118.pdf.
2. Jeff Valentine, "Measuring and Assessing Study Quality," Presentation for The Campbell Collaboration, http://www.campbellcollaboration.org/artman2/uploads/1/Quality_Assessment_Valentine_2013.ppt.pdf.
3. "Grades of Recommendation," The JBI Approach (Joanna Briggs Institute, 2014), http://joannabriggs.org/jbiapproach.html#tabbed-nav=Grades-of-Recommendation.
4. https://cerqual.org.
5. "Levels of Evidence," The JBI Approach (Joanna Briggs Institute, 2014), http://joannabriggs.org/jbiapproach.html#tabbed-nav=Levels-of-Evidence.

stakeholders and audience of the systematic review report. Authors should consider consumers/patients, practitioners, fellow researchers, funders, policy makers, and the public (Booth, Sutton, and Papaioannou 2016). This will be more fully discussed in chapter 10. The *Cochrane Handbook*, section 12, provides guidance on this step as well, describing how to interpret statistical results as well as implications for practice and research (Higgins, Green, and Cochrane Collaboration 2008). While Cochrane's standards call for authors to provide implications for research with standard C80, standard C79 discourages authors from making recommendations as "local considerations may be relevant" (Chandler et al. 2013).

TEXTBOX 9.2. EXPLANATION OF RESULTS

- What are the patterns in the data?
- What is the gap in the literature? What is still unknown?
- What are the strengths of the review?
- How does it compare to other previous reviews?
- What are the implications of the synthesis?
- What are the limitations of the systematic review? What is the likelihood that potential studies were missed?

CONCLUSION

While the planning, identifying, and evaluating steps establish the bones of the review, collecting, combining, and explaining are the heart of the systematic review, and summarizing brings it all together. Librarians can participate in these steps by providing resources through links, articles, tutorials, and books. In addition, librarians may consider learning more about these steps through training to be able to collaborate more thoroughly in all of the processes in the review method.

REFERENCES

Baxter, Susan K., Lindsay Blank, Helen Buckley Woods, Nick Payne, Melanie Rimmer, and Elizabeth Goyder. 2014. "Using Logic Model Methods in Systematic Review Synthesis: Describing Complex Pathways in Referral Management Interventions." *BMC Medical Research Methodology* 14:62. doi:10.1186/1471-2288-14-62. http://www.ncbi.nlm.nih.gov/pubmed/clipboard.

Booth, Andrew, Diana Papaioannou, and Anthea Sutton. 2012. *Systematic Approaches to a Successful Literature Review*. Los Angeles: Sage.

Booth, Andrew, Anthea Sutton, and Diana Papaioannou. 2016. *Systematic Approaches to a Successful Literature Review*. 2nd ed. Los Angeles: Sage. https://study.sagepub.com/booth2e.

Buscemi, N., L. Hartling, B. Vandermeer, L. Tjosvold, and T. P. Klassen. 2006. "Single Data Extraction Generated More Errors than Double Data Extraction in Systematic Reviews." *Journal of Clinical Epidemiology* 59 (7): 697–703.

Chandler, J., R. Churchill, J. Higgins, T. Lasserson, and D. Tovey. 2013. *Methodological Standards for the Conduct of New Cochrane Intervention Reviews*. Cochrane Collaboration.

Cooper, Harris M., Larry V. Hedges, and Jeff C. Valentine. 2009. The Handbook of Research Synthesis and Meta-Analysis. New York: Russell Sage Foundation.

Dixon-Woods, Mary. 2011. "Using Framework-Based Synthesis for Conducting Reviews of Qualitative Studies." *BMC Medicine* 9:39. doi:10.1186/1741-7015-9-39.

Elamin, M. B., D. N. Flynn, D. Bassler, M. Briel, P. Alonso-Coello, P. J. Karanicolas, et al. 2009. "Choice of Data Extraction Tools for Systematic Reviews Depends on Resources and Review Complexity." *Journal of Clinical Epidemiology* 62 (5): 506–10. doi:10.1016/j.jclinepi.2008.10.016.

Gough, David, Sandy Oliver, and James Thomas. 2012. *Introduction to Systematic Reviews*. Los Angeles: Sage.

Gough, David, James Thomas, and Sandy Oliver. 2012. "Clarifying Differences between Review Designs and Methods." *Systematic Reviews* 1:28. doi:10.1186/2046-4053-1-28.

Heyvaert, M., B. Maes, and P. Onghena. 2013. "Mixed Methods Research Synthesis: Definition, Framework, and Potential." *Quality & Quantity* 47 (2): 659–76. doi:10.1007/s11135-011-9538-6. http://search.proquest.com/docview/1271879698.

Higgins, J. P., Sally Green, and Cochrane Collaboration. 2008. *Cochrane Handbook for Systematic Reviews of Interventions*. Chichester, England; Hoboken, NJ: Wiley-Blackwell.

Jonnalagadda, S. R., P. Goyal, and M. D. Huffman. (2015). "Automating Data Extraction in Systematic Reviews: A Systematic Review." *Systematic Reviews* 4 (1): 78. doi:10.1186/s13643-015-0066-7.

Kastner, M., J. Antony, C. Soobiah, S. E. Straus, and A. C. Tricco. 2016. "Conceptual Recommendations for Selecting the Most Appropriate Knowledge Synthesis Method to Answer Research Questions Related to Complex Evidence." *Journal of Clinical Epidemiology* 73:43–49.

Kicinski, Michal, David A. Springate, and Evangelos Kontopantelis. 2015. "Publication Bias in Meta-Analyses from the Cochrane Database of Systematic Reviews." *Statistics in Medicine* 34 (20): 2781–93. doi:10.1002/sim.6525.

Kneale, Dylan, James Thomas, and Katherine Harris. 2015. "Developing and Optimising the Use of Logic Models in Systematic Reviews: Exploring Practice and Good Practice in the Use of Programme Theory in Reviews." *PloS One* 10 (11): e0142187. doi:10.1371/journal.pone.0142187. http://www.ncbi.nlm.nih.gov/pubmed/clipboard.

Lewin, Simon, Claire Glenton, Heather Munthe-Kaas, Benedicte Carlsen, Christopher J. Colvin, Metin Gülmezoglu, Jane Noyes, Andrew Booth, Ruth Garside, and Arash Rashidian. 2015. "Using Qualitative Evidence in Decision Making for Health and Social Interventions: An Approach to Assess Confidence in Findings from Qualitative Evidence Syntheses (GRADE-CERQual)." *PLoS Medicine* 12 (10): e1001895. doi:10.1371/journal.pmed.1001895. http://www.ncbi.nlm.nih.gov/pubmed/26506244.

Li, Tianjing, S. Swaroop Vedula, Nira Hadar, Christopher Parkin, Joseph Lau, and Kay Dickersin. 2015. "Innovations in Data Collection, Management, and Archiving for Systematic Reviews." *Annals of Internal Medicine* 162 (4): 287–94. doi:10.7326/M14-1603.

Mao, Zhi, Lihai Zhang, Yaolong Chen, and Peifu Tang. 2013. "GRADE Outcomes or Studies: How to Use the GRADE Approach Correctly." *International Orthopaedics* 37 (3): 553. doi:10.1007/s00264-012-1766-4. http://www.ncbi.nlm.nih.gov/pubmed/clipboard.

Shea, B. J., J. M. Grimshaw, G. A. Wells, M. Boers, N. Andersson, C. Hamel, A. C. Porter, P. Tugwell, D. Moher, and L. M. Bouter. 2007. "Development of AMSTAR: A Measurement Tool to Assess the Methodological Quality of Systematic Reviews." *BMC Medical Research Methodology* 7:10.

Wilson, D. B. 2009. "Systematic Coding" in *Handbook of Research Synthesis.* Cooper, H. M., Larry V. Hedgers, and Jeffrey C. Valentine, eds. New York: Russell Sage Foundation.

Chapter Ten

Summarizing

Writing Review Protocols and Reports

Mary Lou Klem and Charles Wessel

There is not a discovery in science, however revolutionary, however sparkling with insight, that does not arise out of what went before.

—Isaac Asimov from *Adding a Dimension*

OBJECTIVES

- Provide an overview of the history and nature of reporting guidelines
- Describe the summary documents generated for a systematic review
- List the information elements of a summary document that may be provided by a librarian
- List methods for keeping up to date with systematic review reporting guidelines

OVERVIEW

The final step of the review process is to bring all of the pieces together in a summary report, which may vary in format, but the intent remains the same—to disseminate the results and place the findings into the context of previous studies. Reports of research study methods and findings should be clear, thorough, and transparent so that a reader will be able to replicate the study, interpret the data, apply the results, and understand the study's strengths and weaknesses. Far too often authors omit key information through selective reporting of outcomes, nonreporting or delayed reporting of whole studies, omission of crucial detail about study methodology, omissions or misrepresentation of results in abstracts, and inadequate or distorted reporting of harms (Simera et al. 2010). These problems are not limited to reports of original research—evaluations of published systematic reviews have also found poor and inadequate reporting (Moher et al. 2007; Roundtree et al. 2009; Samaan et al. 2013).

Reporting guidelines are documents designed with the intent of assisting authors in writing and documenting essential elements of a proposed or completed research study. Reporting guidelines are typically developed through a consensus process, usually by an international multidisciplinary group, and are disseminated through publication in well-known professional journals. A more recent trend has been the publication of guidelines in open access journals (Moher et al. 2010) and/or via a free-standing website, such as http://www.consort-statement.org, http://www.prisma-statement.org, http://www.strobe-statement.org, or http://www.squire-statement.org.

Reporting guidelines exist for many different study types, such as case reports, controlled trials, or systematic reviews, and all share common elements. Those elements address the information to include in the title and abstract, introduction, methods, results, and discussion. Additional elements address information specific to the study type. For example, a guideline for case reports (Gagnier et al. 2013) stipulates that such reports should include clinical findings such as medical and family history, pertinent comorbidities, and the results of physical examinations.

A reporting guideline often consists of several different documents, including a reporting statement, an elaboration and explanation document, a checklist, and a flowchart or flow diagram. The purpose of these documents is to guide authors in reporting a specific type of research, developed using explicit methodology (Moher et al. 2010).

The reporting statement typically provides an outline of all the recommended reporting elements. The elaboration and explanation document lists each reporting element and provides a rationale and the evidence base (if any) for the element, as well as an example on how to report that element. A checklist is a one-page document that can be used to indicate if all elements are reported and can be submitted along with the manuscript for publication by a journal. A flowchart or flow diagram is used within the manuscript itself to illustrate a critical study process from start to end. For instance, a flow diagram for a report of a randomized controlled trial illustrates the movement of potential and actual participants through the trial, and a flow diagram for a systematic review graphically represents the flow of article citations and full-text articles through screening for inclusion in the final review.

It is important to keep in mind that the recommendations in reporting guidelines are not rules and that not all reporting guidelines have been adopted by journal publishers (Stevens et al. 2014). Even when adopted, journals may selectively choose the elements for which they mandate adherence (Golub and Fontanarosa 2015).

Brief History of Reporting Guidelines

One of the first reporting initiatives was a proposal to adopt a structured approach for items to be reported in a manuscript abstract (Ad Hoc Working Group for Critical Appraisal of the Medical Literature 1987). The intended purpose of this structured abstract was to "facilitate peer review before publication, assist clinical readers to find articles that are both scientifically sound and applicable to their practices, and allow more precise computerized literature searches" (Haynes et al. 1990). The structured abstract was endorsed and adopted by the International Committee of Medical Journal Editors (International Committee of Medical Journal Editors 1993). Recent library literature continues to follow the adoption of structured abstracts (Hartley 2014; Nakayama et al. 2005; Ripple et al. 2011).

Other early efforts to enhance research reporting focused on guidance provided by journal editors on items to be included when reporting clinical trials (Altman and Simera 2015). Inadequate reporting of randomized controlled trials led to the simultaneous development of reporting guidelines (Standards of Reporting Trials Group 1994; Working Group on Recommendations for Reporting of Clinical Trials in the Biomedical Literature 1994). The two groups leading these initiatives later coalesced to develop a single reporting guideline for randomized controlled trials, the well-known CONsolidated Standards Of Reporting Trials (CONSORT) Statement (Begg et al. 1996).

The CONSORT Statement and Checklist provide details of twenty-five required reporting items for a clinical trial. These evidence-based reporting items include a description of the trial's design, data, and results, as well as a flow diagram illustrating how participants proceeded through the trial. The CONSORT statement is endorsed by almost six hundred journals and two major organizations for journal editors, the International Committee of Medical Journal Editors (ICMJE) and the World Association of Medical Editors (WAME) (CONSORT Group 2010). Numerous studies have evaluated the use of the CONSORT statement and its checklist and have found better trial reporting and improved reporting compliance in trials published in CONSORT endorsed journals (Plint et al. 2006; Samaan et al. 2013; Turner et al. 2012). Compliance to CONSORT continues to be examined by specific disciplines with most noting that reporting has improved along with suboptimal adoption of the guidelines (Edwards et al. 2015; Munter et al. 2015; Sandhu, Sandhu, and Kaur 2015). The CONSORT Statement is routinely updated and extended to reflect current clinical trial methodology, including how to report different types of data (harms, abstracts), designs (pragmatic trials, cluster trials), and interventions (herbal medicinal, nonpharmacologic treatments) (CONSORT Group 2012). The CONSORT Statement has become the model for the development of many other reporting guidelines, including those for systematic reviews and meta-analyses (Warner 2013).

The Quality of Reporting of Meta-Analyses (QUOROM) conference was held in 1996 to address reporting of meta-analyses of randomized controlled trials (Moher et al. 1999). In 1997, the Meta-Analysis of Observational Studies in Epidemiology (MOOSE) working group was formed to address reporting of observational studies in meta-analyses (Stroup et al. 2000). Both the QUOROM statement and the MOOSE Statement include a reporting checklist and flow diagram illustrating the number of studies initially identified by the literature search, studies included or excluded in the meta-analysis, and reasons for exclusion (Institute of Medicine 2008). In 2009, QUOROM was replaced by the Preferred Reporting Standards for Systematic Reviews and Meta-Analyses (Liberati et al. 2009).

Additional Reporting Guidelines

The majority of published reporting guidelines are designed for use with reports of biomedical or health sciences literature. However, guidelines are available for other disciplines and subspecialties, including psychology, general education, engineering education, behavioral medicine, and animal research (Borrego, Foster, and Froyd 2014; Cooper 2011). Table 10.1 shows the variety of guidelines available for reporting discipline- or topic-specific research.

Librarians and Reporting Standards

Librarians work diligently to improve scholarly communication, and reporting guidelines can be a major component in this process. Even though editors, funding bodies, peer reviewers, and readers benefit when reporting guidelines are followed, adherence to and adoption of reporting guidelines by journal publishers is far from adequate (Stevens et al. 2014). Librarians can help make researchers and students aware of the existence of reporting guidelines and explain why thorough reporting is beneficial (Golub and Fontanarosa 2015; Leeflang 2015; Moher et al. 2015). When reporting guidelines are adopted, individuals involved in the publication cycle benefit in the ways shown in textbox 10.1 (Leeflang 2015; Samaan et al. 2013).

Table 10.1. Diversity of discipline-specific reporting guidelines

Organization/discipline	*Reporting guideline*
American Educational Research Association	Standards for Reporting on Empirical Social Science Research (American Educational Research Association 2006) Standards for Reporting on Humanities-Oriented Research (American Educational Research Association 2009)
American Psychological Association	Journal article reporting standards (JARS) (APA Publications and Communications Board Working Group on Journal Article Reporting Standards 2008)
Animal research	Animal Research: Reporting In Vivo Experiments (The ARRIVE Guidelines) (Kilkenny et al. 2010)
Behavioral medicine	WIDER recommendations for reporting of behavior change interventions (Albrecht et al. 2013)
Education	Reporting of Primary Empirical Research Studies in Education (The REPOSE Guidelines) (Newman and Elbourne 2004)
Public health	Transparent Reporting of Evaluations with Nonrandomized Designs (TREND) statement (Des Jarlais, Lyles, and Crepaz 2004)
Software engineering	Guidelines for conducting and reporting case study research in software engineering (Runeson and Höst 2009)

TEXTBOX 10.1. BENEFITS OF REPORTING GUIDELINES

- Authors—use guidelines for study planning and reporting, resulting in a manuscript that maximizes transparency and reproducibility
- Editors—guidelines enhance the reporting quality of submitted manuscripts; able to use reporting checklists as part of the editorial policy
- Peer reviewers—can use reporting checklists to assess manuscript and study quality
- Funding agencies—guidelines enhance the quality of funded research projects
- Institutional review boards—ensure that studies are of sound methodological quality
- Librarians—to help access the literature when providing clinical information
- Readers—provides a guide for determining if a study is applicable to the situation they are in

It is important to realize that current reporting guidelines may change over time and that new reporting guidelines will likely be developed in the future. Table 10.2 lists online resources that may be helpful in keeping up to date with reporting guidelines for both quantitative and qualitative research, as well as disciplines outside the health sciences.

It may also be useful to check with coauthors to determine if they are aware of reporting guidelines for their topic or discipline, to search the websites of major professional organizations or journals, or to search the World Wide Web for existing or emerging reporting guidelines (try exercise in action box 10.1).

Table 10.2. Online resources for finding reporting guidelines

EQUATOR (Enhancing the QUAlity and Transparency Of health Research) Network, http://www.equator-network.org	The EQUATOR Network provides free resources and tool kits for users of reporting guidelines, as well as a free database of reporting guidelines. Also offers a newsletter and calendar of upcoming classes and training.
National Library of Medicine's Research Reporting Guidelines and Initiatives, https://www.nlm.nih.gov/services/research_report_guide.html	Based on content from the EQUATOR Network, this charts lists major biomedical research reporting guidelines.
Medline/PubMed Research Reporting Guidelines Search, https://www.nlm.nih.gov/services/guidelinesearch.html	This executable search filter, designed for use in PubMed, finds citations of published reporting guidelines.
PLOS Collections: Reporting Guidelines, http://collections.plos.org/reporting-guidelines	A collection of open access reporting guidelines, as well as discussion of the importance of such guidelines and evidence supporting their use.
The Joanna Briggs Institute, http://www.joannabriggs.org	Supports the design and conduct of research synthesis and dissemination, focusing on comprehensive reviews of topics of interest to the social sciences and humanities, utilizing qualitative, economic, or policy research.
The Campbell Collaboration, http://www.campbellcollaboration.org	Produces systematic reviews on topics related to crime and justice, education, international development, and social welfare. They offer free access to templates for systematic review protocols and manuscripts.

ACTION BOX 10.1

Search Google Scholar to identify discipline-specific reporting guidelines with the following search string: "reporting guideline":"reporting guidelines":"reporting standard":"reporting standards."

SYSTEMATIC REVIEWS AND REPORTING GUIDELINES

Conducting versus Reporting

Existing systematic review guidelines can be divided into those that address all aspects of the systematic review process, from establishing a review team to preparation and publication of a final report, and those that address solely the reporting of a proposed or completed review. Examples of the former include the *Methods Guide for Effectiveness and Comparative Effectiveness Reviews* (Agency for Healthcare Research and Quality 2014), *Cochrane Handbook for Systematic Reviews of Interventions* (Higgins and Green 2011), *Joanna Briggs Institute Reviewers' Manual* (Joanna Briggs Institute 2014), and *Systematic Reviews: CRD's Guidance for Undertaking Reviews in Health Care* (Centre for Reviews and Dissemination 2009). The most comprehensive guidance for both conducting and reporting systematic reviews is found in *Finding What Works in Health Care: Standards for Systematic Reviews* (Institute of Medicine 2011). Published in 2011, this National Academies report utilizes expert guidance from other published standards, as well as available empirical evidence (Institute of Medicine 2011), to create an extensive set of recommendations for designing, conducting, and reporting systematic reviews of comparative effectiveness research. In the spirit of transparency, the report includes a series of tables that display each standard and the corresponding elements of guidance from other standards that served as the basis for that National Academies standard (Institute of Medicine 2011).

Reporting Documents Generated for a Systematic Review

Reporting the details of a systematic review can begin well before the start of the review process itself, through the publication of a review protocol. A protocol specifies in advance a review's proposed methodology and is a document long required by well-known sponsors or producers of systematic reviews, for example, the Cochrane Collaboration. Creation of a protocol requires the review team to think carefully about their approach to the review, to create detailed procedures and data management strategies, and, most importantly, to avoid arbitrary decision making that may introduce bias into study results or synthesis (Shamseer et al. 2015). Results of a completed systematic review may be reported in abstract or manuscript form. Authors seeking to present their results at a professional conference typically submit only an abstract and then, if chosen to present, elaborate on that abstract in a poster or paper format. Results of the review may also be submitted for publication in a journal; in that case, both an abstract and a complete manuscript will be developed.

PRISMA: Preferred Reporting Items for Systematic Reviews and Meta-Analyses

The most well-known guideline for producing various formats and stages of the review is PRISMA: Preferred Reporting Items for Systematic Reviews

TEXTBOX 10.2. PRISMA GUIDELINE AND GUIDELINE EXTENSIONS

- PRISMA Statement
    - PRISMA Statement
    - PRISMA Explanation and Elaboration
    - PRISMA checklist
    - PRISMA flow diagram
- Extensions
    - PRISMA for Abstracts
    - PRISMA Equity
    - PRISMA Harms (for reviews including harm outcomes)
    - PRISMA Individual Patient Data
    - PRISMA for Network Meta-Analyses
    - PRISMA for Protocols
- Extensions in development
    - Preferred Reporting Items for Systematic Reviews and Meta-Analyses—for Children (PRISMA-C)
    - Preferred Reporting Items for Systematic Reviews and Meta-Analyses—Protocols for Children (PRISMA-PC)
    - PRISMA-DTA: Preferred Reporting Items for Systematic Reviews and Meta-Analyses of Diagnostic Test Accuracy Studies

and Meta-Analyses (Moher et al. 2009). It has undergone several edits, translations, and extensions, including a guide for writing a protocol and a guide for abstracts of systematic reviews. A list of PRISMA guides is detailed in box 10.2.

Published in 2009, PRISMA is a revision of the QUOROM statement (Moher et al. 1999). The PRISMA Statement consists of a brief narrative about the history and process of revising QUOROM, a PRISMA checklist (a list of information to be provided when reporting a systematic review or meta-analysis), and a flow diagram for depicting the flow of information through the systematic review process. A separate article, the PRISMA Explanation and Elaboration statement (Liberati et al. 2009), provides for each of the twenty-seven PRISMA checklist items a rationale for including each item as well as examples of good reporting of items. The PRISMA group subsequently published additional documents that provide guidance for the writing of systematic review protocols (Moher et al. 2015; Shamseer et al. 2015), conference and article abstracts (Beller et al. 2013), reports of reviews that utilize individual participant data or focus on health equity (Stewart et al. 2015; Welch et al. 2012), and flowcharts for updates of Cochrane systematic reviews (Stovold et al. 2014).

The PRISMA Statement and PRISMA Explanation and Elaboration articles were published simultaneously in *PloS Medicine*, the *Annals of Internal Medicine*, and other high-profile biomedical journals. Numerous journals subsequently endorsed the PRISMA Statement, agreeing to require inclusion of a completed PRISMA checklist and flow diagram in any systematic reviews or meta-analyses submitted for publication (PRISMA Group 2015). PRISMA standards form the basis of the reporting standards in *Finding What Works in Health Care* (Institute of Medicine 2011) and are incorporated into a new edition of systematic review standards from the Cochrane Collaboration (Chandler et al. 2013). Given this widespread adoption, the PRISMA statement and related documents should be considered gold standards for reporting either a proposed or completed systematic review.

It is important to note two caveats about the PRISMA guidelines. First, PRISMA guidelines are for the reporting of systematic reviews of studies evaluating health-care interventions (Liberati et al. 2009). Thus certain elements of the guidelines may not be applicable for other types of comprehensive literature reviews, or for reviews on topics other than health-care interventions. Authors of such reviews, however, may still benefit from the use of PRISMA guidelines by including relevant elements in their manuscripts or abstracts and excluding those that are clearly inappropriate (Moher et al. 2015). Second, PRISMA guidelines are only for reporting a planned or completed systematic review—they are not designed to serve as "how to" guides on the design and conduct of such projects. Individuals seeking to develop and complete a high-quality review should consult resources specifically focused on conceptualization and design of systematic reviews, such as *Finding What Works in Health Care* (Institute of Medicine 2011) or the *Cochrane Handbook for Systematic Reviews of Interventions* (Higgins and Green 2011), and if possible should recruit a team member with expertise in systematic review methods (Institute of Medicine 2011). Further, it should be emphasized that reporting guidelines such as PRISMA enhance the transparency of a project but provide no guarantee that the review was conducted in a rigorous manner (Schulz, Moher, and Altman 2014). That is, author adherence to a reporting guideline such as PRISMA provides reviewers and readers with information needed to make judgments on the overall quality of the completed review but is not a substitute for those judgments.

Reporting Elements: The Details

This section focuses on selected PRISMA reporting elements (for a protocol, abstract, or journal article) that are most likely to be the responsibility of a librarian, or that would benefit from input from a librarian. The selected elements are listed and discussed below, and a brief summary is also available (librarian's corner 10.1). Unless otherwise noted, all recommendations or explanations are from articles published by Moher et al. (2009), Liberati et al. (2009), Beller et al. (2013), Moher et al. (2015), and Shamseer et al. (2015).

TEXTBOX 10.3. DESCRIBING THE SEARCH STRATEGY

"We searched the following databases: Ovid MEDLINE, including in-process and other nonindexed citations, from 1950 to April 2012 in week 1; Ovid Embase from 1980 to 2012 in week 14; the Cochrane Database of Systematic Reviews, Cochrane CENTRAL Registry of Controlled Trials, and National Health Service Economic Evaluations Databases, through the Wiley interface, through April 16, 2012. The original search was completed November 2010 and was updated April 16, 2012. There were no language or study design restrictions applied to the search (eAppendix 1). The search was peer reviewed through the Peer Review of Electronic Search Strategies Forum. In addition, we contacted researchers to obtain additional data, when applicable."

JAMA Pediatrics. 2013. 167 (3): 259–65. doi:10.1001/2013.jamapediatrics.216.

While this section focuses on a subset of PRISMA reporting elements, librarians will likely benefit from reading and being familiar with all published PRISMA reporting standards, including the helpful "real life" examples of section content provided in PRISMA explanation and elaboration statements (Beller et al. 2013; Liberati et al. 2009; Shamseer et al. 2015). This additional information may be particularly helpful during the final review of a protocol or manuscript prior to submission to a research registry or journal.

Coauthorship

A librarian who designs and conducts literature searches for a systematic review has made a substantive scholarly contribution to the project and, as such, should serve as a coauthor (International Committee of Medical Journal Editors 2016). All authors on the protocol or manuscript should provide basic contact information, including name, institutional affiliation, and e-mail address, and the document should indicate the contributions of each author. Interestingly, the original PRISMA statement did not stipulate that author contributions be defined—that item is found only in the PRISMA guideline for protocols. However, it is increasingly common for journals to request (and in some cases require) that published articles provide details on author contributions, so inclusion of this information in the final manuscript, as well as the protocol, would be wise. Descriptions of each author's contribution(s) are typically very short, no more than one to two brief sentences (see Shamseer et al. 2015, page 4, for an example).

Eligibility Criteria

A systematic review protocol will include a detailed description of the study and report characteristics to be used as inclusion and exclusion criteria. Study characteristics include the patient population of interest, intervention(s) and comparison groups, and outcome variables of interest, while report characteristics include language of publication, publication status, and dates of publication. An abstract should contain only a brief summary of the study and report characteristics used, as well as any date limitations and the inclusion (or not) of studies published in languages other than English. In a final manuscript, the eligibility criteria section elaborates and expands upon the abstract's information and typically includes a rationale for utilizing certain criteria, e.g., lack of access to translation services led to exclusion of non-English language studies. It is likely that the primary author on the protocol or manuscript will be responsible for writing most of the eligibility criteria section, for either a protocol or manuscript. However, the librarian or information specialist designing and conducting the literature search may be responsible for application of one or more criteria, for example, by designing a search that limits dates of publication or article language, and so should check the draft and final copy of the protocol, abstract, or manuscript to ensure that these criteria are included.

Information Sources

It is strongly recommended that the librarian on the review team offer to write this section, as well as the section on search strategies (see below), either during the initial reference interview with team members or at any time when discussing or negotiating project roles and responsibilities. It is likely that colleagues will be more than happy to allow a librarian to take the lead on writing these important sections, and doing so will decrease the likelihood that revisions or editing of these sections will be required during final review of the protocol or manuscript. The importance of designing the search strategy and the need for extensive documentation, discussed in chapter 5, becomes clear when writing up sections for the review protocol or completed report.

For a review protocol, this section should include a list of the bibliographic databases that will be searched, as well as the platform for each database—for example, EBSCOhost—and the date range that will be covered by the search. Discussion of database selection is beyond the purview of this chapter (see chapter 5), but there is consensus that for most biomedical topics, a search of Medline and additional subject-specific databases is a minimum requirement (Higgins and Green 2011; Institute of Medicine 2011).

In addition to the databases to be searched, this section will describe any other sources or search methods that will be used to identify potential studies, including grey literature sources (chapter 6). The name of each source should be provided, as well as the date range that will be searched. If, for example, hand searching will be used, the protocol should specify the titles of journals that will be hand searched and the publication dates that will be included. This section should also describe any searching that does not use a formal information source, for example, scanning of reference lists from included articles, contact with topic experts or authors of included articles, or searches of personal article collections.

A conference abstract or abstract for a final manuscript will contain only limited information about the sources searched. If three or fewer bibliographic databases were searched, the names of each should be provided. If more than three were searched, the abstract should list only the names of the three databases that provided the majority of included studies. The date ranges searched, or the date of the last search, should also be reported. Importantly, note that the abstract does not need to include search platform names, other sources (such as grey literature), or other search strategies.

For the final manuscript, the information sources section will expand upon the basic information provided in the abstract. As in the protocol, all databases (and their search platforms) should be listed, as well as dates of coverage for each database, and the period of time included in the search strategy (if different from database coverage). The date of the last search, or the time period during which all searches were run, should also be provided. Finally, this section should provide detailed descriptions of any additional sources or search strategies that were used, providing source names and dates of coverage as appropriate.

Search Strategy

Begin with a short narrative description of the overall approach to search development. This description will list the name of each database to be searched, including search platform and database coverage. Identify who is responsible for the search and the qualifications of that individual, as well as the topic concepts that form the basis of the search term harvesting (see chapter 5) and search building. Also indicate if any limits will be applied to the search and, if so, how those limits will be achieved, for example, through use of an available database limit or a search filter. If a search filter will be used, provide evidence of the filter's performance metrics by inclusion of a citation of at least one validation study. Because multiple databases will be searched, briefly describe how the initial search strategy will be adapted or revised for use in those other databases. Plans for updating the searches should be noted as well, with the final manuscript also indicating the period of time covered by the search update. Finally, indicate if the search is to be peer reviewed. If so, include the qualifications of the peer reviewer(s) and the name of any standardized assessment instrument used, for example, PRESS (Sampson et al. 2008). While all of this might sound like quite a bit of information, the narrative aspect of a search section can actually be quite short and succinct (see textbox 10.3).

In addition to the narrative, provide readers with a table or appendix that contains, at a minimum, one complete search strategy for one of the major databases (in draft form for a protocol; final form for the manuscript). Copy and paste the search string directly from the database history or a saved search into a table or appendix within the manuscript. The alternative—retyping a search string—only creates opportunities for transcription errors. Finally, note that PRISMA recommends providing a minimum of one search. While including only one (draft) search makes sense for the protocol, consider including

LIBRARIAN'S CORNER 10.1. SUMMARY OF INFORMATION LIBRARIANS TYPICALLY PROVIDE FOR SYSTEMATIC REVIEW DOCUMENTS

	Protocol	*Abstract*	*Manuscript*
Author contributions	Author contributions		
Eligibility criteria	Study and report characteristics	Study and report characteristics	Study and report characteristics
Information sources	All intended sources and planned dates of coverage; include grey lit and all other search strategies	Key databases searched (if 3 or fewer, list all; if more than 3, list 3 that provided the majority of included reports); date of last search	All sources searched, dates of coverage, date of last search; identify individual who completed database searches
Search strategy	General approach to search development and qualifications of individual who will conduct searches; draft search for one electronic database		Full search strategy for at least one electronic database
Study selection			Number of database records retrieved; number of records after duplicate removal
Strengths and limitations		Search limits	Search limits; any constraints on access to databases or articles

all final database searches in any manuscript describing a completed systematic review. This provides readers with the most complete understanding of the search process, allowing them to accurately replicate the entire search process.

The PRISMA guidelines for protocols appear to recommend more detailed descriptions of the search strategy than the original PRISMA Statement. Given that any additional information is likely to enhance both the transparency and the replicability of the project, it seems advisable to use the PRISMA protocol search strategy elements to guide writing of both the review protocol and the final manuscript. For conference or journal article abstracts, no information about search strategies needs to be provided.

Study Selection

In this section of the protocol or manuscript, authors must provide a detailed account of how they screened database records and selected full-text articles for data extraction, analysis, and synthesis. Manuscripts of completed systematic reviews (not protocols) should include a PRISMA flowchart to show the logical progression of database records and full-text articles through the study screening process. As the librarian member of the research team, be prepared to provide selected data for the flowchart, typically the number of records identified through database searching, the number of records remaining after removal of duplicates, and the number of citations excluded, depending on the librarian's role.

Limitations and Strengths

The discussion section of an abstract or final manuscript for a completed review should provide readers with information about any aspects of the review process that might limit the validity or generalizability of results. Thus, it is appropriate to note here any application of a language or date of publication limit. It is also important to note any other constraints placed on the search process, such as lack of access to a major bibliographic database or to full-text articles that would have otherwise been included in the review. Fortunately, the discussion section also typically includes mention of the strengths of the completed study. One obvious strength to list is that a librarian or other information specialist designed and completed the literature searches.

Final Review of Protocol, Abstract, or Manuscript

As noted above, a librarian who provides literature search services to a systematic review project has made a substantive contribution to the conceptualization and design of the project (International Committee of Medical Journal

Editors 2016) and should serve as a coauthor on documents arising from the project. In addition to drafting content for the sections outlined above, a librarian coauthor should also read drafts of the entire protocol, abstract, or manuscript, the final complete document before submission for publication, and any subsequent revisions.

CONCLUSION

Librarians can serve a vital role on systematic review teams by staying current with reporting guidelines, making team members aware of existing or new guidelines, and contributing content to review protocols or final manuscripts. Doing so ensures that the librarian's contribution to the project is explained in a way that enhances transparency and allows others to understand and to replicate the literature searches.

REFERENCES

Ad Hoc Working Group for Critical Appraisal of the Medical Literature. 1987. "A Proposal for More Informative Abstracts of Clinical Articles. Ad Hoc Working Group for Critical Appraisal of the Medical Literature." *Annals of Internal Medicine* 106 (4): 598–604.

Agency for Healthcare Research and Quality. 2014. *Methods Guide for Effectiveness and Comparative Effectiveness Reviews*. Rockville, MD: Agency for Healthcare Research and Quality.

Albrecht, L., M. Archibald, D. Arseneau, and S. D. Scott. 2013. "Development of a Checklist to Assess the Quality of Reporting of Knowledge Translation Interventions Using the Workgroup for Intervention Development and Evaluation Research (WIDER) Recommendations." *Implementation Science* 8:52. doi:10.1186/1748-5908-8-52.

Altman, D. G., and I. Simera. 2015. "A History of the Evolution of Guidelines for Reporting Medical Research: The Long Road to the EQUATOR Network." *JLL Bulletin*. Accessed 2015.

American Educational Research Association. 2006. "Standards for Reporting on Empirical Social Science Research in AERA Publications: American Educational Research Association." *Educational Researcher* 35 (6): 33–40.

American Educational Research Association. 2009. "Standards for Reporting on Humanities-Oriented Research in AERA Publications." *Educational Researcher* 38 (6): 481–86.

APA Publications and Communications Board Working Group on Journal Article Reporting Standards. 2008. "Reporting Standards for Research in Psychology: Why Do We Need Them? What Might They Be?" *American Psychologist* 63 (9): 839–51. doi:http://dx.doi.org/10.1037/0003-066X.63.9.839.

Begg, C., M. Cho, S. Eastwood, R. Horton, D. Moher, I. Olkin, R. Pitkin, D. Rennie, K. F. Schulz, D. Simel, and D. F. Stroup. 1996. "Improving the Quality of Reporting of Randomized Controlled Trials: The CONSORT Statement." *JAMA* 276 (8): 637–39.

Beller, E. M., P. P. Glasziou, D. G. Altman, S. Hopewell, H. Bastian, I. Chalmers, P. C. Gotzsche, T. Lasserson, and D. Tovey. 2013. "PRISMA for Abstracts: Reporting Systematic Reviews in Journal and Conference Abstracts." *PLoS Medicine* 10 (4): e1001419. doi:10.1371/journal.pmed.1001419.

Borrego, Maura, Margaret J. Foster, and Jeffrey E. Froyd. 2014. "Systematic Literature Reviews in Engineering Education and Other Developing Interdisciplinary Fields." *Journal of Engineering Education* 103 (1): 45–76. doi:10.1002/jee.20038.

Centre for Reviews and Dissemination. 2009. *Systematic Reviews: CRD's Guidance for Undertaking Reviews in Health Care*. Centre for Reviews and Effectiveness.

Chandler, J., Rachel Churchill, Julian Higgins, Toby Lasserson, and David Tovey. 2013. *Methodological Standards for the Conduct of New Cochrane Intervention Reviews*. Cochrane Editorial Unit.

CONSORT Group. 2010. "CONSORT: Transparent Reporting of Trials." http://www.consort-statement.org.

CONSORT Group. 2012. "Extensions of the CONSORT Statement." http://www.consort-statement.org/extensions.

Cooper, Harris. 2011. *Reporting Research in Psychology: How to Meet Journal Article Reporting Standards*. Washington, DC: American Psychological Association.

Des Jarlais, D. C., C. Lyles, and N. Crepaz. 2004. "Improving the Reporting Quality of Nonrandomized Evaluations of Behavioral and Public Health Interventions: The TREND Statement." *American Journal of Public Health* 94 (3): 361–66.

Edwards, J. P., N. Dharampal, W. Chung, M. S. Brar, C. G. Ball, J. Seto, and S. C. Grondin. 2015. "Has the Quality of Reporting of Randomized Controlled Trials in Thoracic Surgery Improved?" *European Journal of Cardio-Thoracic Surgery*. 49(5): 1476–82. doi:10.1093/ejcts/ezv375.

Gagnier, J. J., G. Kienle, D. G. Altman, D. Moher, H. Sox, and D. Riley. 2013. "The CARE Guidelines: Consensus-Based Clinical Case Reporting Guideline Development." *BMJ Case Reports*. doi:10.1136/bcr-2013-201554.

Golub, R. M., and P. B. Fontanarosa. 2015. "Researchers, Readers, and Reporting Guidelines: Writing between the Lines." *JAMA* 313 (16): 1625–26. doi:10.1001/jama.2015.3837.

Hartley, J. 2014. "Current Findings from Research on Structured Abstracts: An Update." *Journal of the Medical Library Association* 102 (3): 146–48. doi:10.3163/1536-5050.102.3.002.

Haynes, R. B., C. D. Mulrow, E. J. Huth, D. G. Altman, and M. J. Gardner. 1990. "More Informative Abstracts Revisited." *Annals of Internal Medicine* 113 (1): 69–76.

Higgins, Julian P. T., and Sally Green. 2011. *Cochrane Handbook for Systematic Reviews of Interventions*. Version 5.1.0. The Cochrane Collaboration.

Institute of Medicine. 2008. "Appendix D. Standards for Reporting Meta-Analyses of Clinical Trials and Observational Studies: QUOROM and MOOSE." In *Knowing*

What Works in Health Care: A Roadmap for the Nation, ed. Jill Eden, Ben Wheatley, Barbara McNeil, and H. Sox, 199–204. Washington, DC: National Academies Press.

Institute of Medicine. 2011. *Finding What Works in Health Care: Standards for Systematic Reviews*. Washington, DC: National Academies Press.

International Committee of Medical Journal Editors. 1993. "Uniform Requirements for Manuscripts Submitted to Biomedical Journals. International Committee of Medical Journal Editors." *JAMA* 269 (17): 2282–86.

International Committee of Medical Journal Editors. 2016. "Defining the Role of Authors and Contributors." http://www.icmje.org/recommendations/browse/roles-and-responsibilities/defining-the-role-of-authors-and-contributors.html.

Joanna Briggs Institute. 2014. "The Joanna Briggs Institute." Last modified 2014. http://www.joannabriggs.org.

Kilkenny, C., W. J. Browne, I. C. Cuthill, M. Emerson, and D. G. Altman. 2010. "Improving Bioscience Research Reporting: The ARRIVE Guidelines for Reporting Animal Research." *PLoS Biology* 8 (6): e1000412. doi:10.1371/journal.pbio.1000412.

Leeflang, M. M. 2015. "Reporting Diagnostic Accuracy Studies: Where Are We Now?" *Biomarkers in Medicine* 9 (9): 897–99. doi:10.2217/bmm.15.62.

Liberati, A., D. G. Altman, J. Tetzlaff, C. Mulrow, P. C. Gotzsche, J. P. Ioannidis, M. Clarke, P. J. Devereaux, J. Kleijnen, and D. Moher. 2009. "The PRISMA Statement for Reporting Systematic Reviews and Meta-Analyses of Studies That Evaluate Health Care Interventions: Explanation and Elaboration." *PLoS Medicine* 6 (7): e1000100. doi:10.1371/journal.pmed.1000100.

Moher, D., D. J. Cook, S. Eastwood, I. Olkin, D. Rennie, and D. F. Stroup. 1999. "Improving the Quality of Reports of Meta-Analyses of Randomised Controlled Trials: The QUOROM Statement. Quality of Reporting of Meta-Analyses." *Lancet* 354 (9193): 1896–900.

Moher, D., A. Liberati, J. Tetzlaff, and D. G. Altman. 2009. "Preferred Reporting Items for Systematic Reviews and Meta-Analyses: The PRISMA Statement." *PLoS Medicine* 6 (7): e1000097. doi:10.1371/journal.pmed.1000097.

Moher, D., K. F. Schulz, I. Simera, and D. G. Altman. 2010. "Guidance for Developers of Health Research Reporting Guidelines." *PLoS Medicine* 7 (2): e1000217. doi:10.1371/journal.pmed.1000217.

Moher, D., L. Shamseer, M. Clarke, D. Ghersi, A. Liberati, M. Petticrew, P. Shekelle, and L. A. Stewart. 2015. "Preferred Reporting Items for Systematic Review and Meta-Analysis Protocols (PRISMA-P) 2015 Statement." *Systematic Reviews* 4:1. doi:10.1186/2046-4053-4-1.

Moher, D., J. Tetzlaff, A. C. Tricco, M. Sampson, and D. G. Altman. 2007. "Epidemiology and Reporting Characteristics of Systematic Reviews." *PLoS Medicine* 4 (3): e78. doi:10.1371/journal.pmed.0040078.

Munter, N. H., A. Stevanovic, R. Rossaint, C. Stoppe, R. D. Sanders, and M. Coburn. 2015. "CONSORT Item Adherence in Top Ranked Anaesthesiology Journals in 2011: A Retrospective Analysis." *European Journal of Anaesthesiology* 32 (2): 117–25. doi:10.1097/cja.0000000000000176.

Nakayama, T., N. Hirai, S. Yamazaki, and M. Naito. 2005. "Adoption of Structured Abstracts by General Medical Journals and Format for a Structured Abstract." *Journal of the Medical Library Association* 93 (2): 237–42.

Newman, Mark, and Diana Elbourne. 2004. "Improving the Usability of Educational Research: Guidelines for the REPOrting of Primary Empirical Research Studies in Education (The REPOSE Guidelines)." *Evaluation and Research in Education* 18 (4): 201–12.

Plint, A. C., D. Moher, A. Morrison, K. Schulz, D. G. Altman, C. Hill, and I. Gaboury. 2006. "Does the CONSORT Checklist Improve the Quality of Reports of Randomised Controlled Trials? A Systematic Review." *Medical Journal of Australia* 185 (5): 263–67.

PRISMA Group. 2015. "PRISMA: Transparent Reporting of Systematic Reviews and Meta Analyses." http://www.prisma-statement.org.

Ripple, A. M., J. G. Mork, L. S. Knecht, and B. L. Humphreys. 2011. "A Retrospective Cohort Study of Structured Abstracts in MEDLINE, 1992–2006." *Journal of the Medical Library Association* 99 (2): 160–63. doi:10.3163/1536-5050.99.2.009.

Roundtree, A. K., M. A. Kallen, M. A. Lopez-Olivo, B. Kimmel, B. Skidmore, Z. Ortiz, V. Cox, and M. E. Suarez-Almazor. 2009. "Poor Reporting of Search Strategy and Conflict of Interest in Over 250 Narrative and Systematic Reviews of Two Biologic Agents in Arthritis: A Systematic Review." *Journal of Clinical Epidemiology* 62 (2): 128–37. doi:10.1016/j.jclinepi.2008.08.003.

Runeson, P., and M. Höst. 2009. "Guidelines for Conducting and Reporting Case Study Research in Software Engineering." *Empirical Software Engineering* 14 (2): 131–64.

Samaan, Z., L. Mbuagbaw, D. Kosa, V. Borg Debono, R. Dillenburg, S. Zhang, V. Fruci, B. Dennis, M. Bawor, and L. Thabane. 2013. "A Systematic Scoping Review of Adherence to Reporting Guidelines in Health Care Literature." *Journal of Multidisciplinary Healthcare* 6:169–88. doi:10.2147/jmdh.s43952.

Sampson, M., J. McGowan, C. Lefebvre, D. Moher, and J. Grimshaw. 2008. PRESS: Peer Review of Electronic Search Strategies. Canada.

Sandhu, S. S., J. Sandhu, and H. Kaur. 2015. "Reporting Quality of Randomized Controlled Trials in Orthodontics—What Affects It and Did It Improve over the Last 10 Years?" *European Journal of Orthodontics* 37 (4): 356–66. doi:10.1093/ejo/cju050.

Schulz, Kenneth F., D. Moher, and D. G. Altman. 2014. "Ambiguities and Confusions between Reporting and Conduct." In *Guidelines for Reporting Health Research: A User's Manual*, ed. D. Moher, D. G. Altman, Kenneth F. Schulz, Iveta Simera, and Elizabeth Wager, 41–47. Chichester, West Sussex: Wiley Blackwell; BMJ Books.

Shamseer, L., D. Moher, M. Clarke, D. Ghersi, A. Liberati, M. Petticrew, P. Shekelle, and L. A. Stewart. 2015. "Preferred Reporting Items for Systematic Review and Meta-Analysis Protocols (PRISMA-P) 2015: Elaboration and Explanation." *BMJ* 349:g7647. doi:10.1136/bmj.g7647.

Simera, I., D. Moher, A. Hirst, J. Hoey, K. F. Schulz, and D. G. Altman. 2010. "Transparent and Accurate Reporting Increases Reliability, Utility, and Impact of

Your Research: Reporting Guidelines and the EQUATOR Network." *BMC Medicine* 8:24. doi:10.1186/1741-7015-8-24.

Standards of Reporting Trials Group. 1994. "A Proposal for Structured Reporting of Randomized Controlled Trials. The Standards of Reporting Trials Group." *JAMA* 272 (24):1926–31.

Stevens, A., L. Shamseer, E. Weinstein, F. Yazdi, L. Turner, J. Thielman, D. G. Altman, A. Hirst, J. Hoey, A. Palepu, K. F. Schulz, and D. Moher. 2014. "Relation of Completeness of Reporting of Health Research to Journals' Endorsement of Reporting Guidelines: Systematic Review." *BMJ* 348:g3804. doi:10.1136/bmj.g3804.

Stewart, L. A., M. Clarke, M. Rovers, R. D. Riley, M. Simmonds, G. Stewart, and J. F. Tierney. 2015. "Preferred Reporting Items for Systematic Review and Meta-Analyses of Individual Participant Data: The PRISMA-IPD Statement." *JAMA* 313 (16): 1657–65. doi:10.1001/jama.2015.3656.

Stovold, E., D. Beecher, R. Foxlee, and A. Noel-Storr. 2014. "Study Flow Diagrams in Cochrane Systematic Review Updates: An Adapted PRISMA Flow Diagram." *Systematic Reviews* 3:54. doi:10.1186/2046-4053-3-54.

Stroup, D. F., J. A. Berlin, S. C. Morton, I. Olkin, G. D. Williamson, D. Rennie, D. Moher, B. J. Becker, T. A. Sipe, and S. B. Thacker. 2000. "Meta-Analysis of Observational Studies in Epidemiology: A Proposal for Reporting. Meta-Analysis of Observational Studies in Epidemiology (MOOSE) Group." *JAMA* 283 (15): 2008–12.

Turner, L., L. Shamseer, D. G. Altman, K. F. Schulz, and D. Moher. 2012. "Does Use of the CONSORT Statement Impact the Completeness of Reporting of Randomised Controlled Trials Published in Medical Journals? A Cochrane Review." *Systematic Reviews* 1:60. doi:10.1186/2046-4053-1-60.

Warner, Teddy D. 2013. "How to Evaluate Biomedical Research Rigorously." In *The Academic Medicine Handbook: A Guide to Achievement and Fulfillment for Academic Faculty*, ed. Laura Weiss Roberts, 225–32. New York: Springer.

Welch, V., M. Petticrew, P. Tugwell, D. Moher, J. O'Neill, E. Waters, and H. White. 2012. "PRISMA-Equity 2012 Extension: Reporting Guidelines for Systematic Reviews with a Focus on Health Equity." *PLoS Medicine* 9 (10):e1001333. doi:10.1371/journal.pmed.1001333.

Working Group on Recommendations for Reporting of Clinical Trials in the Biomedical Literature. 1994. "Call for Comments on a Proposal to Improve Reporting of Clinical Trials in the Biomedical Literature. Working Group on Recommendations for Reporting of Clinical Trials in the Biomedical Literature." *Annals of Internal Medicine* 121 (11): 894–95.

Chapter Eleven

The Art of Puzzle Solving

Systematic Review Services

Sarah T. Jewell, Margaret J. Foster, and Margaret Dreker

In the nonstop tsunami of global information, librarians provide us with floaties and teach us to swim.

—Linton Weeks

OBJECTIVES

- Describe potential roles for librarians and competencies for participating in systematic review services
- Describe authorship standards
- Describe models of services
- Describe methods to plan a service
- Discuss resources and issues related to developing a service
- List documentation needs of services

OVERVIEW

In a 2013 survey of medical librarians and directors in the United States, 81 percent of directors and 64 percent of librarians reported that some type of service to support systematic reviews was either in place or planned as a future service (Crum and Cooper 2013). Increasingly, standards on systematic review methodology recommend that librarians be involved due to their search expertise, including those from the Cochrane Collaboration, the Campbell Collaboration, and the National Academies (Gore and Jones 2015). Additionally, in a groundbreaking study by Rethlefsen et al., higher-quality search strategies, as evaluated by a modified version of PRESS (Peer Review of Electronic Search Strategies), correlated with librarian involvement in internal medicine systematic reviews (Rethlefsen et al. 2015). It is not so much a question of whether librarians should develop systematic review services to serve their patrons, but a question of how. This chapter addresses that how.

ROLE OF THE LIBRARIAN

Potential Roles

There are a variety of roles a librarian may play in a review, from expert searcher to project leader. In 2003, Beverly, Booth, and Bath described ten roles for information specialists: project leader, project manager, literature searcher, reference manager, document supplier, critical appraiser, data extractor, data synthesizer, report writer, and disseminator. The tasks a librarian takes on in a review will depend on skill levels, clients' needs/requests, and the predefined activities described in service documentation (Beverley, Booth, and Bath 2003).

The typical role and the basis of all other roles is the librarian as the expert searcher. This involves three processes: (1) the research interview, (2) running the search and providing results, and (3) writing up the appropriate sections of the review report. The reference interview (as discussed in chapter 3) is the most challenging step in this process as clients may request help before fully exploring a research question or understanding the process. The librarian may need to help the client in determining the feasibility of the question. Whether this is part of the librarian's role will be determined by the definition of the systematic review service discussed later in this chapter. During the search process, some librarians only conduct searches in the major databases, while other librarians choose to conduct further searches, including grey literature (as discussed in chapter 6), for their clients.

Beyond the typical role, librarians can provide support or participate in the other steps of the review, including screening, appraisal, data abstraction, or analysis. Swinkels described the expanded role as "piloting of inclusion and exclusion criteria on samples of output, identification of quality assessment tools and preparation of public outputs" (Swinkels, Briddon, and Hall 2006). As roles in research projects expand, librarians need to be flexible and sensitive to team dynamics, including workflow preferences and communication (Dudden and Protzko 2011). In addition, librarians can introduce systematic reviews to patrons by providing a general introduction about reviews, what they are and where to find them, and the general process of reviews. As instructors, librarians can develop or participate in courses on systematic

Table 11.1. Potential roles

Role	*Description*	*Steps of the review*
Introductory role	Introduce patrons to systematic review definition and process, locating reviews	Plan
Expert searcher	Codevelop the search strategy and run the searches; also write methodology	Identify
Project management	Creating and updating timetable for project and keeping within budget	All steps
Review leader	Cowriting the initial bid, chairing meetings, cowriting final report, dissemination of findings	All steps
Instructor	Teaching the searching, basics of how to do a systematic review, or complete course on conducting a review	All steps
Methodologist, systematic review methods	Studying and developing best practices for systematic reviews	All steps

reviews. Lastly, as researchers, librarians can investigate systematic review methods to improve the efficiency or validity of various processes.

No matter the level of participation a librarian has in a review project, there are several benefits to both the librarian and the institution. Increasing the collaboration on review projects provides opportunities for interprofessional exchanges between librarians and other professionals. These projects will be more likely to meet standards for completing reviews, as several organizations have added the consulting librarian as part of the process (see librarian's corner 11.1). Librarians' research output increases with authorship on reviews and participation in grant proposals. There is also a potential for additional income as some libraries (and librarians) are being paid for consultations. Lastly, utilization of library services will increase, along with an expanded perspective of what libraries and librarians can offer to researchers (Gore and Jones 2015).

Competencies

In order to fulfill these roles, librarians need to have a variety of competencies depending on the level of involvement. Box 11.1 lists the competencies for the expert searcher role, as well as advanced competencies. While many librarians will already have advanced searching skills, the development of a search for a systematic review is more complicated and requires additional training. The most difficult process of the review is scoping or framing the

LIBRARIAN'S CORNER 11.1. STANDARDS THAT SPECIFY THE NECESSITY OF A LIBRARIAN'S ROLE

Standard	*Librarian role quotation*
Campbell Collaboration	"Methodological expertise includes: information/library science (searching and text retrieval)"
AHRQ "Finding Evidence for Comparing Medical Interventions"	"A librarian or other expert searcher should be involved in the development of the search"
Cochrane Collaboration	"If a [Cochrane Review Group] is currently without a Trials Search Co-ordinator, authors should seek the guidance of a local health-care librarian or information specialist, where possible one with experience of conducting searches for systematic reviews."
Canadian Institutes of Health Research, "Knowledge Synthesis"	"It is strongly recommended that each team includes an expert in the content area(s) covered by the synthesis, an expert in synthesis methods and an information scientist or librarian."
Institute of Medicine, "Finding What Works in Health Care"	Standard 3.1.1 "Work with a librarian or other information specialist trained in performing systematic reviews (SRs) to plan the search strategy."

(Gore and Jones 2015)

question appropriately, which requires plenty of practice to become proficient. The advanced competencies will require training outside of librarianship, such as critical appraisal of research methods and analysis or interpretation of the data (Dudden and Protzko 2011).

Authorship

Authorship for the review should follow standards required for authorship within the discipline of the review. There are a variety of standards for what amount/level of contribution constitutes an author. Box 11.2 provides a quote from the International Committee of Medical Journal Editors (ICMJE) website on the requirements of authorship. Within the standard, the typical role of

TEXTBOX 11.1. COMPETENCIES FOR LIBRARIANS CONSULTING ON SYSTEMATIC REVIEWS

- Competencies to fulfill expert searcher role
  - Overall skills
    - Interaction with clinicians/clients
    - Understand the overall process of systematic reviews
    - Determine the feasibility of a review question
  - Search
    - Develop comprehensive search
    - Hedges of study types
    - Knowledge about databases
    - How to select databases
    - Identify and search other resources
    - Evaluate search and modify appropriately
  - Management
    - Manage articles
    - Document search/retrieval/review
    - Write-up of report
    - Archival processes
- Advanced competencies for roles beyond searching
  - Data management
  - Project management
  - Critical appraisal of research
  - Grant writing
  - Data abstraction

(Dudden and Protzko 2011; Harris et al. 2005; McKibbon 2006)

the librarian as expert searcher meets requirement 1 during the development of the review question, translation of that question into the search strategy, and then implementing that search to acquire the potential articles. Requirement 2 can be met by drafting the appropriate portions within the review report. In the methods section, the search process will be described along with a figure or table with at least one of the actual searches. In the results section, there will be the description of what was retrieved from the searches, de-duplication, and possibly the creation of the PRISMA flowchart. Lastly, in the discussion section, there should be a description of the strengths and limitations of the search, including the estimated potential for the search to have missed articles. Requirement 3 is usually met through the peer-review process, with the journal editor contacting all authors for final approval of the published version. Out of all the requirements, number 4 may be the most difficult, as some reviews may be very clinical or technical and outside the expertise of the librarian.

TEXTBOX 11.2. INTERNATIONAL COMMITTEE OF MEDICAL JOURNAL EDITORS (ICMJE) RECOMMENDED CRITERIA FOR AUTHORSHIP

"Substantial contributions to the conception or design of the work; or the acquisition, analysis, or interpretation of data for the work; AND
Drafting the work or revising it critically for important intellectual content; AND
Final approval of the version to be published; AND
Agreement to be accountable for all aspects of the work in ensuring that questions related to the accuracy or integrity of any part of the work are appropriately investigated and resolved."

Citation: International Committee of Medical Journal Editors. "Defining the Role of Authors and Contributors." Accessed August 7, 2015. http://www.icmje.org/recommendations/browse/roles-and-responsibilities/defining-the-role-of-authors-and-contributors.html.

While the ICMJE standard is influential, it is not consistently followed. Ultimately the responsibility for authorship resides with the group producing the work. The best strategy is to negotiate authorship within the first meeting, as well as to describe policies with the description of the service. The appendix provides an example of a contract that could be signed by researcher(s) and librarian(s) for a review project.

TYPES OF SERVICE MODELS

Before a systematic review service can be launched, the service model must be considered. There are various configurations that can be put into action; it just depends on which model works best for the patrons.

Team Model

Many libraries train multiple librarians in systematic review searching and offer a team of librarians to assist with systematic reviews. One advantage to this approach is that there are a variety of searching perspectives and also peers readily available to peer review search strategies. If one librarian is unavailable, there is usually another available to be assigned to a project. There is potential for specialization to occur among the librarians; for example, perhaps one librarian has more of an expertise in psychosocial systematic reviews, while another might specialize in engineering. There should be a plan in place for how to assign systematic reviews to each librarian ahead of time. Perhaps a supervisor can be in charge of assignments; otherwise, there can be conflict with librarians wanting certain projects or making sure they get a balance of the workload.

A disadvantage of the team approach is that it might be difficult to standardize the type of service that patrons receive. One librarian might be a more experienced searcher than another, or one librarian might prefer to search in Ovid Medline while another prefers PubMed. There can be a working group in order to establish best practices at an institution, but sometimes it is difficult to reach a consensus about certain techniques, and it might be difficult to enforce the search standards. An individual, on the other hand, whose primary assignment is to work with patrons on systematic reviews, can offer consistently excellent service.

Tiered Models

Tiered models of service are becoming common in libraries offering systematic review services. In some cases, there may be a consultation option, while a fee would be required for full service. Delineating services like this can help to weed out groups that are not truly committed to the lengthy process of conducting a systematic review. It can also help to generate income for the library in a time of strained budgets. On the other hand, offering free services to all constituents can be part of a library's mission.

Some tiered models may come about because of a difference in patrons' needs. In academia, the needs of faculty conducting systematic reviews differ from students conducting them. For students, learning how to search databases and manage search results is a part of the learning process, and therefore a librarian may choose to behave in an advisory role for students. Faculty, on the other hand, may be interested in a librarian as a coinvestigator, and the librarian may actually run the searches, collect the results, and de-duplicate them before delivering them to the faculty member.

Case Studies

Boxes 11.3–5 provide examples of libraries providing systematic review services in different ways. As libraries are continuing to build services, some have only one individual offering the service, while others have teams. As systematic review consultations can take a great deal of time and resources, some libraries have selected to charge a fee for the service. These examples provide a quick snapshot of what real libraries are providing right now.

TEXTBOX 11.3. EXAMPLE OF INDIVIDUAL LIBRARIAN–BASED SERVICE

Library: Medical Sciences Library, Texas A&M University, College Station, Texas
Population served: The main groups served are an academic health science center (medicine, nursing, pharmacy, public health, and dentistry), a college of veterinary medicine, agriculture, and a health education program through the College of Education. In addition, any student, faculty, or staff across the university may use the service.
Fee: None
Description: One librarian focuses completely on meeting the needs of systematic review authors across campus. The service provides individual and group consultations on any part of the review process, with authorship negotiated in the initial contact. In addition, class presentations, webinars, and workshops are also offered.
Roles: introductory role, expert searcher, teacher, project manager, review leader

TEXTBOX 11.4. EXAMPLE OF TEAM-BASED SERVICE

Library: Bernard Becker Medical Library, Washington University in St. Louis School of Medicine, St. Louis, Missouri
Clients served: Mostly School of Medicine faculty, staff, researchers, residents, and fellows, also some from the School of Social Work and two teaching hospitals
Fee: None
Description: A team of six librarians led by Susan Fowler, who volunteer to take review requests, handle the systematic review service. Some librarians do specialize in particular areas (e.g., pediatrics).

Authorship is usually granted to the librarians, as they mention it in relation to their writing of the search methodology in their marketing materials, initial meetings, and final e-mails.
Roles: Introductory role, teaching (searching), expert searcher role, conducting these steps: developing and documenting the search in databases, downloading to citation management software and de-duplicating results, and writing the methods section pertaining to the search.

TEXTBOX 11.5. EXAMPLE OF FEE-BASED SERVICE

Library: George T. Harrell Health Sciences Library, Penn State, Hershey, Pennsylvania
Population served: Residents, faculty, and staff of Penn State Milton S. Hershey Medical Center, Penn State College of Medicine, and Penn State Hershey Children's Hospital
Fees: The library charges hourly fees for librarian time based on the individual librarian's compensation (both salary and benefits) and actual hours (cost recovery only). Researchers are also responsible for ILL fees. In addition, library charges fees on a cost-recovery basis for any database searches on systems to which the library does not subscribe (e.g., EMBASE searches).
Description: A team of three librarians (plus one part time). The librarian responsible for oversight of the service determines which librarian will be assigned to a particular review in consultation with the core group and based on expertise and workload. Faculty may also request a specific librarian.
Roles that librarians take: introductory role, teaching (searching), expert searcher role, conducting these steps: developing and documenting the search in databases, downloading to citation management software and de-duplicating results, searching grey literature resources, hand searching if applicable, and writing the methods section pertaining to the search.

PLANNING THE SERVICE

The case studies provided in boxes 11.3–5 offer ideas to help in planning a service, but each service will be unique in order to best serve the needs of the clients and institution. When determining what services should be offered, there are several questions that should be considered (as shown in box 11.6). After considering these questions, the answers could be arranged into a logic model, as shown in table 11.2.

TEXTBOX 11.6. QUESTIONS TO ANSWER WHEN DEVELOPING THE SYSTEMATIC REVIEW SERVICE

- What types of services will be offered?
- Who will be served? What are their needs regarding systematic reviews?
- What librarians/staff will be providing the services?
- Are there resources (time and personnel) available to extend this service?
- What training is needed?
- How will systematic reviews be assigned/allocated?
- Will there be fees?
- What will be required of the client before the meeting?
- How will authorship be considered by the institution and negotiated with clients?

A logic model provides a clear, organized path to move from the aims of a service to the activities and outcomes. First, consider the situation for developing the service, including the issues that led to the development, stakeholders, and their needs. Second, determine the overall aim of the service, including potential challenges and solutions. Next, list the resources that will be needed to meet those aims, and then the outputs (services and deliverables) that will reach those aims. Finally, consider how the service will be evaluated by describing potential measurable outcomes. These outcomes can be listed as short- to long-term goals and should be SMART specific, measurable, action oriented, realistic, and timed.

Table 11.2. Logic model template for developing a service

Rationale	*Aims*	*Resources*	*Outputs*	*Outcomes*
Describe the situation in which the service is developing	Determine the overall goals of service and issues to be resolved	List all resources including staff, funding, training, space, and more	Describe outputs of the service that will meet the aims and be measured by the outcomes	List outcomes which are specific, measurable, action oriented, realistic, and timed
Need that service will meet	Goals	Assets	Activities	Short term
Stakeholders	Challenges or issues	Training needs	Services	Long term
Stakeholder needs	Possible solutions to challenges	Needed resources	Deliverables	Impacts

Source: Adapted from W. K. Kellogg Foundation. 2004. *Logic Model Development Guide*. Battle Creek, MI: W. K. Kellogg Foundation.

Resources and Issues to Consider

Once the service model has been determined, the job description of the librarians involved may need to be updated, or a new job description for a sole systematic review librarian will need to be written. The Medical Library Association website is a good source for sample job descriptions, although delineating which roles a librarian will play in a service also will assist in writing the job description. For librarians working in the library already, adequate time will need to be allocated for systematic review training and the work itself. Lack of time and training are the most frequently reported barriers to a systematic review service, so it is important for managers to recognize the need for both (Murphy and Boden 2015). Some formal level of training should be a prerequisite before a librarian can participate on a systematic review. As for the time needed, one study, which included grey literature as part of the systematic review search process, reported a mean time of almost eight hours and a median time of approximately twenty-four hours for a systematic review search (Saleh et al. 2014).

For funding, whether or not a paid service model is in place, it can become complicated when grants are involved. Some grants may not allow for funding to be spent on a librarian's services, and other times, the library may optimally prefer to become involved during the grant application process to ensure that adequate compensation is allocated to the library for the services rendered.

Additionally, there is some debate in academic circles about whether or not systematic review publications should count toward scholarly publications that are considered during the tenure process. In certain disciplines, systematic review work is not always valued as highly as it should be and is judged as derivative and not original scholarship (Chalmers, Hedges, and Cooper 2002). It may be a challenge for librarians involved with systematic reviews to gain scholarly recognition for their contributions to the field. In the process of developing a systematic review service, it is important to consider issues when demand outpaces the resources available. Librarian's corner 11.2 offers some strategies for dealing with these challenges.

DOCUMENTATION

Documentation can come in two forms: one form that is transparent, for the patron to see, i.e., "front-facing," and another form, which is perhaps more detailed, for the librarian to record search details in like a laboratory notebook, called the "back documentation." In a tiered service model, it is possible that one may use the front-facing documentation for all patrons, but the back documentation only for the more comprehensive level of service.

LIBRARIAN'S CORNER 11.2. STRATEGIES FOR MANAGING A DEMAND FOR LIBRARY SYSTEMATIC REVIEW SERVICES

- Freeing librarians' time by ensuring that all work is appropriately assigned to academic and nonacademic staff
- Building searcher capacity in the librarian community
- Lobbying for additional librarian and expert searcher positions
- Redefining service policies for external users
- Better organizing search support resources
- Negotiating with faculty to make systematic review search assignments reasonable
- Requiring clients to do advance preparation for searches
- Educating our researchers

(Campbell and Dorgan 2015)

To a large extent, documentation is determined by what you plan to report and thus should be guided by PRISMA standards. However, to make the process seamless for patrons, librarians may wish to customize front-facing forms to help guide the patrons through the entire systematic review process. For example, in addition to recording contact information for the patron and librarian, one might include a timeline with blanks for dates, to guide the patron's team in planning their time accordingly. This helps the librarian adjust the patron's expectations as to how long the systematic review might take and establishes deadlines for certain parts of the process.

One might argue that having multiple forms may be off-putting for some patrons, and this depends on the demand for the service. Since systematic reviews are such a big time investment, sometimes it is acceptable to have a barrier in place for the service, so as to weed out patrons not truly serious about the project and to prevent wasted time. There should be space for a PICO to be worked out in the case of medical topics, or for lists of concepts and synonyms of those concepts to be listed in chart form. There should be a space for controlled vocabulary terms to be added.

There should be space for the patron to record certain inclusion/exclusion criteria for the types of documents they will accept. For medical topics, this would include features about the research subjects, such as age, gender, human or animal, nationality, occupation, and geographical setting. For other topics, this would at least include qualities about the documents, such as language, publication date ranges, and types of studies to be included. This can prompt a discussion of different biases that may exist if one places a language limit or date limit on the documents retrieved. This can also lead the way for a discussion of the importance of searching for grey literature and an explanation of what that includes.

A list of databases to be searched is essential for the front-facing documentation. So is deciding upon the format of the results and which citation management software will be used. This can signal to the librarian whether the patron needs training or not in certain software. It can also allow for a discussion of what databases are most appropriate to search for the topic at hand.

One section of the form that is being increasingly included in front-facing forms is a contract-like section. This section can detail the tasks which the librarian will perform, the tasks for which the patron is responsible, whether or not coauthorship will be granted to the librarian, and, finally, even a signature of both librarian and patron, as they enter into an agreement on commencing with the project.

In cases where the librarian is performing the searches and delivering the results to the patron, the back documentation is likely to be more detailed and designed to assist with reporting according to PRISMA guidelines. One must record the name of each database searched, which platform or search interface was used (a technical aspect often missed by patrons but known by librarians to be important), each search strategy in its entirety, and the number of results, alongside the date searched and any limits placed on the search. Additionally, the dates of coverage of each database should be recorded in order to accurately represent the search.

In cases where the librarian is offering comprehensive service, it is recommended that the librarian, who is executing the actual searches, should be the one to write the search methodology section, as this will result in a more accurate reporting. Taking careful notes on the search strategies helps the librarian to craft a well-worded description of the search methods. When recording the search strategies, cutting and pasting the search strategy into a text document is the method preferred by Cochrane. Retyping search strategies is not recommended, as this can introduce errors. In addition to an offline copy of the search strategy saved in a text document, some databases allow search strategies to be saved, which can then be rerun at a later point. Redundancy is desired when recording the search strategies, and for databases which make it difficult to save the search strategy or copy and paste it, it is recommended to take a screenshot of the search as it was run (Rader et al. 2014).

In addition to documenting the search strategies in a text file, saving results as exported text files and saving the records in citation management software is desired. This ensures backup copies of the results in the event that a database is corrupted. It also helps to have the text version of results in the case where the import into citation management software results in missed or mismatched fields. By referring to the text version of the results, it might be possible to clarify details of the citation and obtain missing information.

When saving results in text files, it is recommended to have a naming convention for the files, for example, DatabaseName_N_MMYYYY.txt, where N is the number of results, and MMYYYY is the month and year of the search (Rader et al. 2014).

MARKETING SYSTEMATIC REVIEW SERVICES

Marketing of products in industries is very much essential to increase sales and consequently to gain the profit; however in an academic environment like universities and colleges, promotion and marketing of the library and information sector is required to be aware of the library services (Patil and Pradhan 2014). Marketing is a systematic approach to identifying specific user needs, providing services to meet these needs, and persuading users of the need to act. The focus is on matching customers with quality services through community involvement. This is an ongoing process that anticipates the need for change.

The main segmentations of library marketing are the users. In an academic medical library, this includes students, faculty, staff, researchers, and general library users. It can be difficult to work out a single marketing strategy that reaches all segments of users. Many times it is worthwhile to formulate different strategies for individual user groups. "The strategies a library uses to market its expertise may affect the number of researchers requesting librarian assistance as well as how researchers perceive librarians as systematic review collaborators" (Ludeman et al. 2015).

Library marketing research has experienced a shift from selling the library toward meeting the needs of users (Weingand 1999). Effective marketing requires careful planning, creative approaches, and focused strategies. Researchers are often unaware of the skills and expertise of the librarians. Efforts to raise awareness therefore need to include not only the marketing of library products (e.g., databases), but also the expertise of the librarians in information seeking (e.g., systematic reviews), information organizing (e.g., research data management), and skills to enable access to information (e.g., nonprint materials, grey literature, special collections, and archives) and preservation. By getting involved in their own research, librarians will further be able to not only demonstrate more advanced research skills but will also be able to engage with researchers on a higher level.

The best marketing tool in promoting a systematic review service is to achieve some quick wins. In other words, do some little marketing things that work well and bring back instant results—this makes everyone more positive and less distrustful about the skills of the librarians on the systematic review team. And then shout about the results from the rooftops! You need buy-in from everyone for library marketing to work well.

One of the main goals of marketing this service is to be able to assess behavior. For marketing to work really well, you need to actually change people's behavior as a result of your efforts—Are they asking for librarian assistance? Are they completing a form asking for a meeting with the librarian about systematic reviews? And so forth.

E-mail announcements sent to faculty and students at each school, on each campus is an effective way to reach a large audience at one time. It can be targeted more precisely than most other methods and so is effective at reaching specific audiences. By maintaining up-to- date address lists, different user groups can be targeted with different versions of the advertising. Systematic review services for students may differ from services offered for faculty members. Targeted e-mail can address this to each population.

"A banner across the library's homepage, and an article in the library's bi-monthly newsletter" is another way to advertise this new library service (Ludeman et al. 2015). A library homepage serves as a promotional tool advertising new library services and electronic information resources. The pages should include an e-mail link to the systematic review service web page making the librarian easy to contact.

Social media such as blogs, e-newsletters, YouTube, Facebook, Twitter, and podcasts are free and easy ways to introduce the new service. An assessment of their effectiveness should be done to see if these methods are reaching your target audience.

Sometimes marketing a service is not a tangible thing. It is personalized service that is adapted to fit an individual or a team's needs. You need to be professional and use quality procedures, but you also need to smile and establish a personal relationship with as many of your users as possible. Establish the key players and the people who can and want to help. Word of mouth marketing is still the best marketing a library service can benefit from. You need champions for each area—satisfied customers who will spread the word among their peers. If you can get bosses on your side, they can even talk about using the systematic review service in the library as a commitment to improve research.

LibGuide or Website Guides

Librarians have encountered a wide range of background knowledge among researchers requesting systematic reviews. Many have no prior experience conducting systematic reviews and have limited knowledge of the scope of the project (Ludeman et al. 2015). Having prepared handouts or web-based materials to outline the systematic review process can be very helpful to clarify the process and time commitment before beginning.

LibGuides, a SpringShare web-based content management and publishing system is one way to do this. The LibGuide can be used to promote the systematic review service. It can share web-based media such as videos, and link to documents and other tutorials to explain the systematic review process and the service offered in the library. The Memorial Sloan Kettering Library and many others offer this form of guidance to its users (https://library.mskcc.org). The LibGuide offers information on the systematic review service and can help manage expectations of users. The LibGuide also offers contact information directly to the systematic review librarian for more assistance.

Example of Website

The George F. Smith Library of the Health Sciences at Rutgers University has a web page (shown in action box 11.1) that offers entrance to a portal which differentiates between librarian services for students or for faculty. The portal has information about the systematic review process, a timeline of the research, a breakdown of responsibilities of each member of a review team, and a form to set up a meeting with a librarian to clarify any question the user may have.

ACTION BOX 11.1. EXAMPLE OF WEBSITE DESCRIBING A SERVICE

Visit the Systematic Reviews Service page of the George F. Smith Library of Health Sciences, part of Rutgers, State University of New Jersey, at http://www.libraries.rutgers.edu/health_sciences/SRS.

INSTRUCTIONAL SESSIONS

Running instructional and informational sessions on the systematic review process for potential users can help overcome gaps in that knowledge. Gatherings that outline the systematic review process can be presented at lunch time "brown-bag" workshops, at grand rounds, or at other departmental sessions.

There are many opportunities in an academic medical library to introduce the importance of librarians' involvement in the systematic review process. This would include presentations in faculty orientations and grand rounds.

Exposing students to the service during a class orientation is another way to address your targeted users.

Having a librarian liaison working with the university research office is another avenue for "selling" the systematic review service. Researchers may be more willing to include a librarian on the systematic review team when they understand the specialized knowledge and skills the librarian can bring to the process.

As librarians we should be actively marketing and promoting our library services. The basic aim of marketing is to know and understand our users in order that the library will be able to satisfy those needs in an effective way. A marketing plan is an essential tool which will enable us to focus our efforts. The marketing plan should assess where you are now (market research), where you are going (objectives), and how you are going to get there (strategies). This may also mean measuring marketing success and making modifications.

It is gratifying to contribute to the development of important new standards, policies, and practices and to be recognized for the range of skills and expertise librarians bring to the effort (Dudden and Protzko 2011). Creating online tools and sending print or e-mail materials is a good start, but it's only part of the equation. The other part is engaging with systematic review service users to let them know their librarians can be a valuable part of the systematic review team. Effective and honest communication with researchers is still the best marketing for this service.

CONCLUSION

Librarians have a vital role in introducing patrons to reviews, conducting systematic reviews, teaching, and researching systematic review methods. All of these roles will require additional training and striving to keep up with the latest standards, improvements to methods, and opportunities for funding and publishing. Clearly defining the service, including negotiating authorship, will lead to better outcomes for patrons and librarians. While offering a service requires a commitment of time and resources, the resulting research output will benefit all involved.

REFERENCES

Beverley, C. A., A. Booth, and P. A. Bath. 2003. "The Role of the Information Specialist in the Systematic Review Process: A Health Information Case Study." *Health Information and Libraries Journal* 20 (2): 65–74.

Campbell, Sandy, and Marlene Dorgan. 2015. "What to Do When Everyone Wants You to Collaborate: Managing the Demand for Library Support in Systematic Review Searching." *JCHLA/JABSC* 36:1119.

Chalmers, I., L. V. Hedges, and H. Cooper. 2002. "A Brief History of Research Synthesis." *Evaluation & the Health Professions* 25 (1): 12–37.

Crum, J. A., and I. D. Cooper. 2013. "Emerging Roles for Biomedical Librarians: A Survey of Current Practice, Challenges, and Changes." *Journal of the Medical Library Association: JMLA* 101 (4): 278–86.

Dudden, R. F., and S. L. Protzko. 2011. "The Systematic Review Team: Contributions of the Health Sciences Librarian." *Medical Reference Services Quarterly* 30 (3): 301–15.

Gore, Genevieve C., and Julie Jones. 2015. "Systematic Reviews and Librarians: A Primer for Managers." *Partnership: The Canadian Journal of Library & Information Practice & Research* 10 (1): 1–16.

Harris, M. R. 2005. "The Librarian's Roles in the Systematic Review Process: A Case Study." *Journal of the Medical Library Association*: JMLA 93 (1): 81–87.

International Committee of Medical Journal Editors. "Defining the Role of Authors and Contributors." Accessed August 7, 2015. http://www.icmje.org/recommendations/browse/roles-and-responsibilities/defining-the-role-of-authors-and-contributors.html.

Ludeman, E., K. Downton, A. G. Shipper, and Y. Fu. 2015. "Developing a Library Systematic Review Service: A Case Study." *Medical Reference Services Quarterly* 34 (2): 173–80.

McKibbon, Ann. 2006. "Systematic Reviews and Librarians." *Library Trends* 55 (1): 202–15. doi:10.1353/lib.2006.0049.

Murphy, S. A., and C. Boden. 2015. "Benchmarking Participation of Canadian University Health Sciences Librarians in Systematic Reviews." *Journal of the Medical Library Association: JMLA* 103 (2): 73–78.

Patil, S. K., and Pranita Pradhan. 2014. "Library Promotion Practices and Marketing of Library Services: A Role of Library Professionals." *Procedia: Social and Behavioral Sciences* 133:249–54.

Rader, T., M. Mann, C. Stansfield, C. Cooper, and M. Sampson. 2014. "Methods for Documenting Systematic Review Searches: A Discussion of Common Issues." *Research Synthesis Methods* 5 (2): 98–115.

Rethlefsen, M. L., A. M. Farrell, L. C. Osterhaus Trzasko, and T. J. Brigham. 2015. "Librarian Co-Authors Correlated with Higher Quality Reported Search Strategies in General Internal Medicine Systematic Reviews." *Journal of Clinical Epidemiology* 68 (6): 617–26.

Saleh, A. A., M. A. Ratajeski, and M. Bertolet. 2014. "Grey Literature Searching for Health Sciences Systematic Reviews: A Prospective Study of Time Spent and Resources Utilized." *Evidence Based Library & Information Practice* 9 (3): 28–50.

Swinkels, A., J. Briddon, and J. Hall. 2006. "Two Physiotherapists, One Librarian and a Systematic Literature Review: Collaboration in Action." *Health Information and Libraries Journal* 23 (4): 248–56.

Weingand, Darlene E. 1999. *Marketing and Planning Library and Information Services*. Englewood, CO: Libraries Unlimited.

Chapter Twelve

The Last Piece

Librarianship and Systematic Reviews

Margaret J. Foster and Sarah T. Jewell

The medical literature can be compared to a jungle. It is fast growing, full of deadwood, sprinkled with hidden treasure and infested with spiders and snakes.

—Peter P. Morgan. *Canadian Medical Association Journal* (Morgan 1986)

OBJECTIVES

- Describe additional ways librarians can contribute to systematic reviews
- Describe common barriers in completing reviews
- Discuss emerging techniques in systematic review methods
- Provide overview of librarianship and reviews

OVERVIEW

Librarians are well equipped to be guides through the ever-increasing jungle of literature, no matter the field. With this book, we aim to equip our readers with tools sharp as a machete to cut a path through to the best evidence. However, the jungle is always growing, and thus we conclude with ways librarians can have an ever-increasing role in collaborating and producing systematic reviews. As systematic review methods continue to evolve, researchers and practitioners work to advance concepts, guides, standards, software, and other resources. Librarians can participate in these endeavors, adding their own experiences, perspectives, and unique set of skills.

THE INTERSECTION OF LIBRARIANS AND SYSTEMATIC REVIEWS

Librarians have a variety of ways that they can contribute to systematic review utilization, creation, and methods (see librarian's corner 12.1). As an individual librarian learning about reviews, one can continue to increase participation as understanding and skills increase. First, librarians can encourage students, researchers, and practitioners to seek and appraise systematic reviews as potential sources of information. Next, librarians can offer their searching skills during the identifying stage of the reviews, eventually moving into other steps of the review with experience. In addition, librarians can join the effort to develop software and other resources for the challenges faced by review authors. Lastly, librarians can engage in producing systematic reviews on topics of interest in the practice of librarianship and research in information science. Each of these roles can be enhanced by participating in professional development, collaborating with researchers on projects, and sharing with other librarians through professional organizations.

LIBRARIAN'S CORNER 12.1. ACTIVITIES FOR LIBRARIANS IN SYSTEMATIC REVIEW METHODS

- Develop and validate search filters or hedges
- Participate or lead in the development standards for review methods
- Design software or other tools for reviews
- Create tutorials and other resources for systematic review authors
- Serve as peer reviewer for searches of review protocols or review reports under consideration for publication
- Develop new techniques for improving the efficiency of citation searching, retrieval, de-duplication, or selection
- Track potential opportunities for funding systematic reviews
- Join grant proposal teams and funded research

LIBRARIAN AND INFORMATION SCIENCE PROFESSIONAL ORGANIZATIONS

The Medical Library Association's activities reflect those of its members in systematic reviews. In 1992, Schell and Rathe published one of the first articles detailing the ways a librarian could participate in a systematic review (Schell and Rathe 1992). Over the years, several continuing education courses were offered providing training on how to consult on a review. The MLA Research Section developed a research agenda which called for volunteer groups to answer fifteen questions with systematic review methods (Eldredge et al. 2012). Then, in 2014, the Systematic Reviews Special Interest Group was founded which offers a forum to communicate and learn with others. Other library organizations are just beginning to join in, such as American College and Research Libraries (ACRL). In 2013, an article in ACRL proceedings described systematic reviews as a research collaboration opportunity for librarians (Monroe-Gulick, O'Brien, and White 2013). In 2016, a short article on systematic reviews was published in the current awareness publication *Keeping Up With . . .* by ACRL (Thomas 2016). Many of the endeavors and proposals by the professional organizations were aimed at discussing and educating about offering a systematic review service within libraries.

SERVICES IN LIBRARIES: MEETING THE CHALLENGE OF CONDUCTING SYSTEMATIC REVIEWS

Since systematic reviews are often performed by novices to the process, librarians play an important role in training these researchers and in identifying common barriers and issues. Some of the largest stumbling blocks to researchers performing systematic reviews have been studied in software engineering (Carver et al. 2013). According to the survey responders, the most time-consuming aspects include extracting the data and selecting papers, followed by searching the databases and assessing the quality. In addition, the survey showed that the researchers' main need for training focused on searching the databases, with selecting the papers and extracting the data coming in second and third. During the planning step, refining the research question was selected as the most crucial step. Ideally, both a domain expert and a librarian should be consulted in order to scope the question properly. For the identifying step, librarians are helpful in tailoring the search for each database and exporting the results and removing duplicates. Training in how to identify articles according to the inclusion criteria is needed, and so are strategies for resolving conflicting opinions on whether or not particular studies should be included. When assessing the quality of the studies, having an expert review the data extraction form is helpful, and having a librarian to suggest different tools to extract the data (e.g., Covidence, as discussed in chapter 9), or to help develop a form or tool, meets a vital need (Carver et al. 2013).

ADVANCES IN RESOURCES AND TOOLS TO ASSIST WITH REVIEWS

While there are existing systematic review tools available, librarians should have a voice in modifying and developing new tools to meet the needs of researchers. Hassler researched common barriers which could be solved with future tools, describing potential new features in the categories of collaboration, quality assessment, study storage, search and selection, data sharing, and development and validation. Of these categories, the search and selection and collaboration are the most desired tool features. In the search and selection category, semantic searching features are needed, as most current bibliographic databases tend to rely on Boolean operators. A text-mining type of searching could greatly speed the search process and reduce the cognitive load when attempting to translate the research question into a searchable query (Hassler et al. 2016).

Search Filters

One area in which many librarians and information scientists have contributed a great deal is the development and validation of search filters. As discussed in chapter 5, search filters are a search strategy designed for a specific purpose in a specific database. For example, search filters have been designed to retrieve systematic reviews in various databases (e.g., PubMed, Medline, Embase). Most search filters are designed to locate specific types of studies, such as randomized control trials, while others were developed to find studies based on geography, age of participants, and more. Jenkins published a review of search filters in which she described three generations of filters: (1) those subjectively designed, (2) those subjectively designed which are validated with a gold standard set of articles, and (3) those objectively designed and validated with a gold standard (Jenkins 2004). Librarians can participate in the development, appraisal, and validation of search filters. Bak et al. developed a tool to appraise filters, the Canadian Agency for Drugs and Technologies in Health (CADTH) critical appraisal instrument (CAI), which uses nine questions to determine the quality of the filter (Bak et al. 2009). It covers the filter's design, validation test, and limitations.

ACTION BOX 12.1. CRITICALLY APPRAISE A SEARCH FILTER

Find a search filter and use the Canadian Agency for Drugs and Technologies in Health (CADTH) critical appraisal instrument (CAI) to evaluate the filter.

Automation

As technology improves, some processes of the review have been targeted as potential processes to be automated: screening, data extraction, and risk of bias assessment. Several researchers have suggested that the screening process could be automated by using text-mining applications. Text mining is the process of exploring the text to discover and/or organize it. There are two approaches for applying text mining: as a way to classify potential citations as excluded or as a way to order the citations by relevancy. Either of these approaches could benefit from active learning, a technique designed to "teach" the software how to categorize citations (O'Mara-Eves et al. 2015). O'Mara-Eves et al. noted that reordering the citations may not reduce the time to screen articles as reviewers may still choose to manually screen all citations; however, it does allow quick selection of relevant studies so that some of the review team can move on to the next stages. One study of text mining showed that text mining reduced workload by nearly 90 percent (Shemilt et al. 2014). The reliability of text mining is promising in clinical or highly technical disciplines, but less applicable for other disciplines due to the nature of research reports being more vague in other fields.

Data extraction is one of the most time-consuming stages in the systematic review, and some researchers want to improve the efficiency of this step by applying text mining. A 2015 systematic review identified twenty-six reviews which had employed some type of automated data extraction in their process. These reviews crossed several disciplines and were retrieved by searching PubMed, IEEExplore, and ACM Digital Library (Jonnalagadda, Goyal, and Huffman 2015). They found that these reviews extracted in a wide variety of ways, with some only extracting sentences and others extracting data elements. Automated data extraction is still only beginning to be explored but has the potential to lead to living systematic reviews (discussed later in this chapter).

Automating risk of bias has started to be explored in the medical field. Millard, Flach, and Higgins tested a tool that assessed three aspects of randomized control trials (sequence generation, allocation concealment, and blinding). After testing their tool, they concluded that "it is possible to use text mining to reduce the reviewer workload by identifying the articles that have been classified with a certainty higher than that of human reviewers" (Millard, Flach, and Higgins 2016). As critical appraisal is a cornerstone of systematic reviews, this type of tool will need to be validated with further research.

Disseminating and Applying Systematic Reviews

Some other factors to consider are barriers and facilitators to disseminating and applying systematic reviews after they have been published. If the journal or database publishing the systematic review allows or encourages it, providing a one-page summary of main points, including tips for practitioners, is recommended. Use of a graphical representation of the risk of bias, as recommended by the Cochrane Collaboration, can offer a quick judgment of how strong the evidence is. Attempts to contextualize evidence are helpful as well, such as proposing how evidence might be used in different socioeconomic settings. Finally, training practitioners in how systematic reviews can be applied is vital, as sometimes this evidence can be perceived as a cookie-cutter approach to solving problems. Librarians can demonstrate that autonomy in decision making can still be present, even as evidence is used to inform the decision (Tricco et al. 2016).

Updating Reviews

Knowing when and how to update reviews is another issue that arises while collaborating on reviews. Takwoingi et al. note that while the Cochrane Collaboration recommends that systematic reviews be updated every two years, the majority of them are not updated as quickly as this. In order to help prioritize the updating of systematic reviews, they developed a decision tool that involves three questions. The first question asks whether the clinical question remains relevant and whether or not it has already been answered by the available evidence. The second question involves whether any new factors have emerged that could affect the systematic review, such as additional data from included studies, new methodology, feedback to the systematic review, or inclusion in policy decision making or a clinical practice guideline. The final question involves whether any new studies exist, depending on the sample size and number of new studies (Takwoingi et al. 2013). Sutton et al. proposes a method for prioritizing the updating of meta-analyses based on the relative magnitude of the new evidence and the heterogeneity of the studies in order to predict the likelihood of a statistically significant change in the conclusions of a meta-analysis (Sutton et al. 2009).

As there are many organizations involved in funding, conducting, and supporting reviews, it is important to consider policies across organizations. When Garritty et al. carried out an international survey of 127 organizations, only 29 percent were reported to have a written updating policy, and of those, the majority were borrowing the Cochrane Collaboration's policies. Of those considered responsible for updating a systematic review, the authors of the original review, funders, and policy makers using the evidence were considered the most accountable. There is evidence that perhaps librarians need to promote their utility in updating reviews, as information specialists were considered the least responsible for this action. Factors that influenced whether or not a review was updated include a formal request from a policy maker, the number of new studies identified, new evidence that relates to harms and benefits, reporting of new adverse events, time credibility, changes to inclusion criteria, a need for an organization decision, and, finally, the number of participants in the new studies available (Garritty et al. 2010).

Living Systematic Reviews

Systematic reviews can take a long time, and often the date of the last search in a systematic review is over a year ago because of the time it takes to complete the review and go through the peer-review process to be published. Living systematic reviews are a new alternative, and they differ in four ways from a regular systematic review: (1) publication format, (2) work processes, (3) author team management, and (4) statistical methods (Elliott et al. 2014). The publication format is an online-only evidence summary that is updated quickly and often, although the review still undergoes peer and editorial reviews, depending on whether there are new studies updating the review or not. Some suggested places for where these reviews could reside are GitHub and the Systematic Review Data Repository (Badgett et al. 2015). Instead of intense, sporadic work processes, a living systematic review allows for moderate, continuous effort toward updating the review. As far as team management goes, a living review needs to allow for evolution of the team and changes in personnel while maintaining institutional memory. Finally, the recommended statistical method for a living review is a Bayesian framework (Elliott et al. 2014).

Systematic Reviews Applied to Library and Information Science

The application of systematic review methods to library and information science (LIS) related questions provides practitioners, researchers, and policy makers with syntheses. In the past decade, several reviews have been published as well as papers exploring the methods of these reviews. A wiki was developed in 2012 to collect LIS-related systematic reviews which are categorized into topics: reference, education, collections, management, information access and retrieval, professional issues, and knowledge management (Koufogiannakis 2012). The categories with the most reviews (as of July 2016) are reference and information access and retrieval, while the least are collections and management (Koufogiannakis et al. 2015). One issue with the wiki is that some of the listed reviews are not systematic as identified by a methodology review published in 2016 (Maden and Kotas 2016). Despite this issue, the wiki maintains a rich resource for those interested in LIS scholarship.

Several overviews have been published on LIS-related reviews over the years, highlighting various issues. Ankem (2012) identified twelve systematic reviews and meta-analyses by searching library science specific databases (LIS, LISA, and Library Literature) for citations with "systematic review" or "meta-analysis" in the title and selecting only those that were published in a LIS journal by an author who could be identified as affiliated with a library or information center. She noted that all of the included reviews were limited to medical library related topics and had several methodological issues including inadequate clarity of variable definitions and failing to provide a true synthesis. The high level of variation in LIS primary studies contributes to these difficulties.

Maden and Kotas critically evaluated the quality appraisal methods of twenty-six systematic reviews listed in the LIS Systematic Reviews wiki. Their findings highlighted that only 66 percent of the included reviews conducted quality assessments, and only 25 percent considered overall quality of the evidence in the synthesis. The quality assessment tools used by the studies varied widely, with these being two of the most common:

- Twelve-item checklist designed by Booth and Brice for the CRItical Skills Training in Appraisal for Librarians (CriSTAL) project (Booth and Brice 2004), which focused on appraising a user study
- A critical appraisal checklist designed by Glynn to address a broader range of studies as may be encountered by librarians (Glynn 2006)

Maden and Kotas concluded that the lack of standards for systematic reviews within the LIS field has resulted in reviews that are lacking in methodological rigor regarding quality assessment of included studies.

Meta-analyses are one of the most complex forms of synthesis a researcher can endeavor to conduct and have been applied to LIS topics. In 2015, Ke and Cheng published a content analysis of such studies, identifying thirty-five meta-analyses published from 1992 to 2013. The most frequent focus of the studies (twenty-three of thirty-five) was information systems, with such topics as acceptance of technology, adoption issues, and use of information systems (Ke and Cheng 2015). Few studies focused on library reference services or resource management. The authors noted several issues in the application of meta-analysis to LIS topics. First, there is a lack of quantitative studies and reporting of statistics within research studies to make a meta-analysis possible. Second, quality control continues to be an issue, with many studies not reporting homogeneity testing results or searching grey literature. Finally, the term *meta-analysis* has been applied incorrectly (twelve out of forty-seven during the screening phase), which shows a need for guidance and standards for LIS authors.

ACTION BOX 12.2. SYSTEMATIC REVIEW ON LIBRARY SCIENCE TOPIC

Find and critically appraise a systematic review on a library science topic using one of the standard checklists provided in chapter 2 for appraising reviews.

CONCLUSION

When the field of librarianship combines with systematic review methods, the combination provides a rich arena for practice, service, and research of librarians. The interdisciplinary nature and reliance on information management skills of systematic reviews yield an opportunity for libraries to collaborate with researchers in a way not found in most other research methods. While technologies continue to expand the ability to work with larger data sets and automate some of the work in reviews, the need for well-conducted reference interviews and proper planning is where it all starts. Librarians who endeavor to become an indispensable part of the systematic review process will find researchers across disciplines increasingly calling on them to collaborate. By striving to understand each piece of the puzzle, engaging with clients, and advancing systematic review methods, librarians can actively participate in the ever-evolving field of knowledge synthesis.

REFERENCES

Ankem, Kalyani. 2008. "Evaluation of Method in Systematic Reviews and Meta-Analyses Published in LIS." *Library and Information Research* 32 (101): 91–104.

Badgett, Robert G., Mohinder Vindhyal, Jason T. Stirnaman, C. Michael Gibson, and Rim Halaby. 2015. "A Living Systematic Review of Nebulized Hypertonic Saline for Acute Bronchiolitis in Infants." *JAMA Pediatrics* 169 (8): 788–89. doi:10.1001/jamapediatrics.2015.0681. http://www.ncbi.nlm.nih.gov/pubmed/clipboard.

Bak, Greg, Monika Mierzwinski-Urban, Hayley Fitzsimmons, Andra Morrison, and Michelle Maden-Jenkins. 2009. "A Pragmatic Critical Appraisal Instrument for Search Filters: Introducing the CADTH CAI." *Health Information and Libraries Journal* 26 (3): 211–19. doi:10.1111/j.1471-1842.2008.00830.x.

Booth, Andrew, and Anne Brice. 2004. *Evidence-Based Practice for Information Professionals: A Handbook*. London: Facet.

Carver, J. C., E. Hassler, E. Hernandes, and N. A. Kraft. 2013. "Identifying Barriers to the Systematic Literature Review Process." Paper presented at the ACM/IEEE International Symposium on Empirical Software Engineering and Measurement, Baltimore, MD.

Eldredge, Jonathan D., Marie T. Ascher, Heather N. Holmes, and Martha R. Harris. 2012. "The New Medical Library Association Research Agenda: Final Results from a Three-Phase Delphi Study." *Journal of the Medical Library Association: JMLA* 100 (3): 214–18.

Elliott, Julian H., Tari Turner, Ornella Clavisi, James Thomas, Julian P. T. Higgins, Chris Mavergames, and Russell L. Gruen. 2014. "Living Systematic Reviews: An Emerging Opportunity to Narrow the Evidence-Practice Gap." *PLoS Medicine* 11 (2): e1001603. doi:10.1371/journal.pmed.1001603. http://www.ncbi.nlm.nih.gov/pubmed/clipboard.

Garritty, Chantelle, Alexander Tsertsvadze, Andrea C. Tricco, Margaret Sampson, and David Moher. 2010. "Updating Systematic Reviews: An International Survey." *PloS One* 5 (4): e9914. doi:10.1371/journal.pone.0009914.

Glynn, Lindsay. 2006. "A Critical Appraisal Tool for Library and Information Research." *Library Hi Tech* 24 (3): 387–99.

Hassler, E., J. C. Carver, D. Hale, and A. Al-Zubidy. 2016. "Identification of SLR Tool Needs: Results of a Community Workshop." *Information and Software Technology* 70:122–29.

Jenkins, M. 2004. "Evaluation of Methodological Search Filters—a Review." *Health Information and Libraries Journal* 21 (3): 148–63.

Jonnalagadda, Siddhartha R., Pawan Goyal, and Mark D. Huffman. 2015. "Automating Data Extraction in Systematic Reviews: A Systematic Review." *Systematic Reviews* 4:78. doi:10.1186/s13643-015-0066-7.

Ke, Qing, and Ying Cheng. 2015. "Applications of Meta-Analysis to Library and Information Science Research: Content Analysis." *Library & Information Science Research* 37 (4): 370–82.

Koufogiannakis, D., A. Brettle, A. Booth, L. Kloda, and C. Urquhart. 2015. "LIS Systematic Reviews." http://lis-systematic-reviews.wikispaces.com/Welcome.

Koufogiannakis, Denise. 2012. "The State of Systematic Reviews in Library and Information Studies." *Library & Information Science Research* 37 (4): 296–310.

Maden, Michelle, and Eleanor Kotas. 2016. "Evaluating Approaches to Quality Assessment in Library and Information Science LIS Systematic Reviews: A Methodology Review." *Evidence Based Library and Information Practice* 11 (2): 149–76.

Millard, Louise A. C., Peter A. Flach, and Julian P. T. Higgins. 2016. "Machine Learning to Assist Risk-of-Bias Assessments in Systematic Reviews." *International Journal of Epidemiology* 45 (1): 266–77.

Monroe-Gulick, Amalia, Megan S. O'Brien, and Glen W. White. 2013. "Librarians as Partners: Moving from Research Supporters to Research Partners."ACRL Proceedings.

Morgan, P. P. 1986. "Review Articles: Looking Over the Field." *Canadian Medical Association Journal* 134:11–12.

O'Mara-Eves, Alison, James Thomas, John McNaught, Makoto Miwa, and Sophia Ananiadou. 2015. "Using Text Mining for Study Identification in Systematic Reviews: A Systematic Review of Current Approaches." *Systematic Reviews* 4 (1): 1–22.

Schell, C. L., and R. J. Rathe. 1992. "Meta-Analysis: A Tool for Medical and Scientific Discoveries." *Bulletin of the Medical Library Association* 80 (3): 219–22.

Shemilt, Ian, Antonia Simon, Gareth J. Hollands, Theresa M. Marteau, David Ogilvie, Alison O'Mara-Eves, Michael P. Kelly, and James Thomas. 2014. "Pinpointing Needles in Giant Haystacks: Use of Text Mining to Reduce Impractical Screening Workload in Extremely Large Scoping Reviews." *Research Synthesis Methods* 5 (1): 31–49.

Sutton, Alex J., Sarah Donegan, Yemisi Takwoingi, Paul Garner, Carol Gamble, and Alison Donald. 2009. "An Encouraging Assessment of Methods to Inform Priorities for Updating Systematic Reviews." *Journal of Clinical Epidemiology* 62 (3): 241–51. doi:10.1016/j.jclinepi.2008.04.005. http://www.ncbi.nlm.nih.gov/pubmed/clipboard.

Takwoingi, Yemisi, Sally Hopewell, David Tovey, and Alex J. Sutton. 2013. "A Multicomponent Decision Tool for Prioritising the Updating of Systematic Reviews." *BMJ (Clinical Research Ed.)* 347: f7191. http://www.ncbi.nlm.nih.gov/pubmed/clipboard.

Thomas, C. 2016. "Keeping Up with . . . Systematic Literature Reviews." *Keeping Up with* . . . . http://www.ala.org/acrl/publications/keeping_up_with/slr.

Tricco, A. C., R. Cardoso, S. M. Thomas, S. Motiwala, S. Sullivan, M. R. Kealey, B. Hemmelgarn, et al. 2016. "Barriers and Facilitators to Uptake of Systematic Reviews by Policy Makers and Health Care Managers: A Scoping Review." *Implementation Science* 11 (1).

Appendix

Rutgers Biomedical Health Sciences (RBHS) Libraries Systematic Review Services

Section 5: Tasks
The following tasks must be performed as part of a systematic review. Please let us know which of these tasks you would like a librarian to perform.

***Note: If you wish a librarian to perform the tasks in bold, the librarian will be included as a coauthor of the published study.*

_____ Check for existing or ongoing systematic reviews on the same topic.
_____ ***Design the systematic review search strategy.***
_____ Send a copy of the first 100 citations from Medline to the SR team and consult about the search.
_____ ***Run searches in appropriate databases.***
_____ Arrange for peer review of the search strategy (add one week).
_____ Support grey literature search.
_____ Create an EndNote library with all retrieved results and remove duplicates.
_____ **Compile a flow diagram of the selection process (the research team must provide this data).**
_____ Prior to final write-up, rerun Medline search strategy to retrieve new studies.
_____ Write the sources and search methodology section.
_____ Final review of the article.
_____ EndNote training for the team.

Section 6: Agreement
Please read this agreement and sign below.
The librarian will provide a signed copy for you.

The team leader and the contact person understand that a *minimum of two months* from the date of the agreement are required for delivery of the work done by the librarian (not including flow diagram and methodology). If a shorter time frame is required, the search is treated as a comprehensive search and not considered systematic—the search will not be peer reviewed, and only one or two databases will be searched.

The team leader, the contact person, and the librarian agree to the estimated time frame for delivery of the work done by the librarian, **with the understanding that any time estimates are subject to change depending on the nature and complexity of the search, and that factors out of the control of the librarian (technical problems with databases) may impact on the estimated timeline**.

The team leader and the contact person agree to answer all communication in a timely manner in order to facilitate completion of the librarians' work within the estimated time frame. **The contact person should be available to answer questions within two business days.**

The **librarian will be named as coauthor on the final publication**. The librarian will also be assured that their contribution to the review will not be altered unless there is a discussion with the team leader.

Signature of Team Leader ______________________ Date ________________

Signature of Contact Person ____________________ Date ________________

Signature of Librarian __________________________ Date ________________

If possible please e-mail this completed form to Systematic Review Service or srsearch@libraries.rutgers.edu.

Index

Page references for figures are italicized.

About the Editors and Contributors

Margaret J. Foster, MS, MPH, AHIP, is an associate professor at Texas A&M University and serves as the systematic reviews coordinator at the Medical Sciences Library with joint positions at the School of Public Health and the College of Medicine. Focusing on systematic reviews for the past decade, she has consulted on hundreds of reviews across a variety of disciplines, published articles on applying or describing systematic review methods, provided training for over four hundred librarians, and founded the Medical Library Association Systematic Review Special Interest Group.

Sarah T. Jewell, MLIS, with over a decade of experience in science and medical libraries, has been instrumental in launching two systematic review services, one at the Memorial Sloan Kettering Cancer Center Library and another at Rutgers University Libraries. She has coauthored many systematic reviews with various research teams, and is pleased to share her expertise in this area. She serves as a newsletter coeditor for the NY-NJ Medical Library Association chapter, is a column editor for the *Journal of Hospital Librarianship*, and also conducts peer reviews for the *Annals of Family Medicine*.

* * *

Nancy J. Allee, MLIS, MPH, AHIP, is deputy director, Taubman Health Sciences Library, University Library, and library faculty, Department of Learning Health Sciences, Medical School. She is a member of the Academy of Health Information Professionals at the distinguished level and serves on the editorial boards of the *Journal of the Medical Library Association* and *Medical Reference Services Quarterly*, is an editorial advisor to *Evidence Based Library and Information Practice*, and is one of the managing assistant editors for a new open access journal, *Learning Health Systems*. She teaches an MLA (Medical Library Association) continuing education course, Planning, Conducting, and Publishing Library Research, and has participated on MLA and medical education systematic review project teams.

Margaret Rush Dreker, MPA, MLS, has been on the staff of the George F. Smith Library of the Health Sciences of Rutgers University since 2001. She has an MPA from New York University and an MLS from Rutgers University. Margaret has worked with faculty and students completing systematic reviews for over ten years.

Erin Eldermire, MLIS, head of the Flower-Sprecher Veterinary Library at Cornell University, received her MLIS from Syracuse University after ten years as a wildlife biologist. In 2015, she and her colleagues launched a systematic review service to support non-medical disciplines at Cornell University. Through this service, she supports nontraditional systematic reviews in agriculture, the life sciences, and related fields. Her broad interests lie in making interdisciplinary connections to spark discovery and collaboration and breaking down barriers for scholarship and research.

Susan A. Fowler, MLIS, is the library director at Washington University Brown School: Social Work and Public Health. Her current interests include creating reporting standards for systematic review search strategies and finding a pragmatic solution for search strategy peer review. Susan has coauthored several published systematic reviews, a book chapter on designing effective search strategies for nurses conducting systematic reviews, and a column on information resources in the *American Journal of Nursing*.

Mary Lou Klem, PhD, MLIS, has been a research and instruction librarian at the University of Pittsburgh Health Sciences Library System for eleven years. She has served as library liaison to the University of Pittsburgh School of Nursing for the past ten years and is one of the founding instructors for the HSLS Systematic Review Workshop: The Nuts and Bolts for Librarians. Prior to becoming a librarian, Dr. Klem was an assistant professor of psychiatry in the University of Pittsburgh School of Medicine.

Mark P. MacEachern, MLIS, is an informationist at the University of Michigan A. Alfred Taubman Health Sciences Library. He teaches within the dental and medical school curricula and frequently partners and consults with researchers on systematic review projects. He coordinates the University of Michigan's flipped systematic review course, Systematic Reviews: Opportunities for Librarians.

Misa Mi, PhD, MLIS, MA, AHIP, is an associate professor in the Department of Biomedical Sciences of the Oakland University William Beaumont School of Medicine and a librarian at the medical library of the medical school. She has over twenty years of experience working in different library settings and developing and teaching training programs in evidence-based medicine, systematic reviews, critical appraisal of systematic reviews, information management, and curriculum development. She has authored numerous peer-reviewed journal articles, book chapters, and other types of scholarly work. She has an MLIS and PhD from Wayne State University, an MA from Oakland University, and received her training in the Program for Educators in the Health Professions from the Harvard Macy Institute, Harvard University.

Heather K. Moberly, MSLS, AHIP, AFHEA, is the coordinator of veterinary services at the Medical Sciences Library at Texas A&M University with a joint appointment in the College of Veterinary Medicine and Biomedical Sciences. She focuses on veterinary professional and graduate education, particularly evidence-based veterinary medicine. Beyond the university curriculum, she bridges the information and veterinary worlds by developing and teaching continuing education to both librarians and veterinarians. She travels extensively, presenting information about locating and incorporating information into veterinary practice. Additionally, she holds the Dorothy G. Whitley Professorship in Library Science where her research focuses on the literature of veterinary parasitology and collaborative evidence-based veterinary medicine education.

Julie H. Schiavo, MLIS, AHIP, is an assistant librarian and head dental librarian at Louisiana State University Health Sciences Center, New Orleans. She received her MLIS from the University of Southern Mississippi and a Certificate of Advanced Studies in Health Science Librarianship from the University of Pittsburgh. She is a distinguished member of the Academy of Health Information Professionals. Julie is a certified reviewer for the Joanna Briggs Institute and coordinates the systematic review service at the LSUHSC-NO Libraries.

Jenni Simonsen, MBA, MSLS, earned her MBA (agribusiness specialty) from New Mexico State University and her MSLS from Clarion University of Pennsylvania. Previously a research specialist at New Mexico State University where her research explored marketing and consumer preference issues affecting agriculture, she began her career in librarianship as an agriculture and life sciences librarian at Texas A&M University. Most recently, she was strategic assessment projects librarian at Texas A&M's Medical Sciences Library.

Elizabeth Stellrecht, MLS, is a senior assistant librarian for the Health Sciences Library at the University at Buffalo. Liz serves as the clinical librarian and liaison to the School of Dental Medicine and assists faculty, staff, and students with their research needs. As clinical librarian, she spends a portion of her week embedded in the dental outpatient clinics to support evidence-based patient care.

Whitney A. Townsend, MLIS, has been an informationist at the University of Michigan A. Alfred Taubman Health Sciences Library since 2007. In addition to teaching in the medical school curriculum, she works with clinical and research faculty in multiple departments to integrate evidence-based information into clinical practice. Whitney partners with many faculty on systematic review projects and coteaches the flipped-classroom workshop Systematic Reviews: Opportunities for Librarians.

Charles B. Wessel, MLS, joined the Health Sciences Library System (HSLS)—University of Pittsburgh in 1986. Over the years his roles have included user education and literature searching for University of Pittsburgh Medical Center (UPMC) clinicians, clinical medical librarian for general internal medicine morning report and the palliative care team rounds, and management of hospital library services and access services. His current role is head of research initiatives where he participates as a coinvestigator on systematic review and other study design teams. He chairs the HSLS Systematic Review Group and is a member of HSLS's management committee. For his digital vitae, go to http://www.hsls.pitt.edu/about/staff/profile?name=cbw.

Sarah Young, MS, MSSc, MLIS, is a liaison librarian at Carnegie Mellon University. She served as the health sciences librarian at Cornell University's Albert R. Mann Library from 2012 to 2016, providing reference, instruction, and research support for students and researchers in nutritional sciences, human development, and policy analysis and management. She holds advanced degrees in biology and international development and an MLIS from the University of Pittsburgh. Since 2013, Sarah has provided systematic review support to researchers in global and public health among other disciplines and served as teaching faculty in the annual WHO/Cochrane Collaboration/Cornell University Summer Institute for Systematic Reviews in Nutrition for Global Policy Making.

www.ingramcontent.com/pod-product-compliance
Ingram Content Group UK Ltd.
Pitfield, Milton Keynes, MK11 3LW, UK
UKHW012038150926
475560UK00001B/67

9 781442 277014